Fritz Jahr

Essays in Bioethics 1924 – 1948

Ethik in der Praxis/Practical Ethics

Materialien/Documentation

herausgegeben von

Hans-Martin Sass
Ruhr-Universität Bochum,
Potomac Institute for Policy Studies,
Arlington VA

Schriftleitung: Arnd T. May

Band 15

LIT

Fritz Jahr

Essays in Bioethics 1924 – 1948

Edited and translated by Irene M. Miller and Hans-Martin Sass

LIT

Supported by a Grant of the Zentrum fuer Medizinische Ethik, Bochum

Bibliographic information published by the Deutsche Nationalbibliothek
The Deutsche Nationalbibliothek lists this publication in the Deutsche Nationalbibliografie; detailed bibliographic data are available in the Internet at http://dnb.d-nb.de.

ISBN 978-3-643-90337-2

A catalogue record for this book is available from the British Library

Klosbachstr. 107
CH-8032 Zürich
Tel. +41 (0) 44-251 75 05
Fax +41 (0) 44-251 75 06
E-Mail: zuerich@lit-verlag.ch
http://www.lit-verlag.ch

LIT VERLAG Dr. W. Hopf
Berlin 2013
Fresnostr. 2
D-48159 Münster
Tel. +49 (0) 2 51-62 03 20
Fax +49 (0) 2 51-23 19 72
E-Mail: lit@lit-verlag.de
http://www.lit-verlag.de

Distribution:
In Germany: LIT Verlag Fresnostr. 2, D-48159 Münster
Tel. +49 (0) 2 51-620 32 22, Fax +49 (0) 2 51-922 60 99, E-mail: vertrieb@lit-verlag.de

In Austria: Medienlogistik Pichler-ÖBZ, e-mail: mlo@medien-logistik.at
In Switzerland: B + M Buch- und Medienvertrieb, e-mail: order@buch-medien.ch
In the UK: Global Book Marketing, e-mail: mo@centralbooks.com
In North America: International Specialized Book Services, e-mail: orders@isbs.com
e-books are available at www.litwebshop.de

TABLE OF CONTENT

Articles by Fritz Jahr

UNIVERSAL LANGUAGE AND THE LANGUAGES OF THE WORLD. 1924

The universal language movement as a whole has taken on such proportions that it cannot be overlooked any longer, provided one chooses not to overlook it. Also, the practical application is larger than it would appear to the casual observer. It is no wonder then, that the one or other universal language has found entrance in schools here or there, a development that pleases the overseeing authorities. Therefore, it seems only right and proper, that teaching staffs of all schools should show an interest in this movement, if only for the sake of taking a pro or con position. To be able to take a proper position, one must gain certain knowledge of potential problems and their history. This requires far more than could be offered in a short essay. An especially important and little known fact needs to be pointed out, the universal language movement is not identical with Esperanto. There is not only one single universal language, but there are several.

The mistaken view, that only a single universal language exists, and that it is Esperanto, is widespread. In reality several universal languages coexist, besides Esperanto, e.g. Esperantita, Ido, Interlingua and Occidental, and these systems, besides, are not as insignificant as would appear. Take for example Ido, a reformed Esperanto, which was created by an academy of scholars and practitioners within a five year span from 1907-1912. Ido, as well, is known the world over. e.g., it is taught at the Prag Handelsakademie. Soviet Russia has also accepted Ido. A strong Ido movement exists as well in labor at home and abroad. It is also widespread within civil society. We have e.g., a Catholic Ido Society. As a consequence the Prussian Minister for Teaching, the Arts and

Community Education [Minister für Unterricht, Kunst und Volksbildung] wants to incorporate Ido advancement. Ido is already being taught in schools especially in the Anhalt. – Esperanto is still the most common among the universal languages, as it is the oldest. Is it by no means the only one, yes; it has found an equal in Ido.

Esperanto is not the only universal language; it is also the least complete. This becomes evident when comparing it to the other systems, especially the Ido. Esperanto, in comparison with the last mentioned language, takes the place of the older, less developed, while Ido is younger and on a higher step. Ido is marked especially by its greater simplicity, naturalness, precision, and beauty. – We find a further difference in that the originator of Esperanto, the Polish-Jewish physician Zamenhof, did not wish his creation to be submitted to further development, which all living languages must undergo. Further, he regarded his universal language as fundamentally unchangeable and stiff. This aspect brings with it an aging and outdating of Esperanto, until finally it becomes useless, unless it already has succumbed to splintering. Indeed, already now it is no longer a unified language. In contrast, Ido is principally designed for development, but it is a planned, instead of random development. It is directed by an academy of suitable scholars and practitioners, similar to the *Academy Française* for the French language, and gives Ido a similar and greater significance. In this way it is possible to keep Ido abreast of all future new cultural developments, as well as avoidance of splintering and safeguarding its unity of development. – Finally, Esperanto lacks scientific interaction, save some casual association. Ido, in contrast, is in well organized and close association with same. – Prof. Wilhelm Ostwald, keeping these and similar facts in view, pronounces judgment in his *"Grundriss der Naturphilosophie"* [Foundation of Natural Philosophy]: "At present, the artificially created language [Hilfssprache] Ido is the most complete realization of a universal language concept". If there be any discussion of a universal language, these words are meant for Ido: "She marches everywhere; she knocks at the gates of your schools. Do you want to welcome her? You will, you can, you want it".

A joint committee of Esperantists and Idoists is presently in formation, to prepare a way of unification of both systems. In view of a global movement of languages, as well as cultures, it would be most advantages, if all universal languages could participate and contribute to its success. In the meantime, no friend of world languages should delay their learning. One may, need be, learn one of their many shorthand systems, even in the hopes of a unified system. It would be most desirable to find many such friends of the universal languages in the national circles, that an original grassroots movement of citizens might not be displaced by political rationalism and thereby discredited.

Weltsprache und Weltsprachen. *Die Mittelschule. Zeitschrift für das gesamte mittlere Schulwesen*, 1926, 44:96-97.
– Jahr's criticism of Esperanto as a stiff and inflexible language is part of an extended discussion in "*Die Mittelschule*", caused by an article by Josef Driesler "Esperanto in der Mittelschule. Selbsterlebtes" [Esperanto in the Middle School. Own Experiences], *Die Mittelschule. Zeitschrift für das gesamte mittlere Schulwesen* 1923, 37(4): 25-28, 33-35.

COMPOSITION AS A METHOD IN TEACHING. 1926

Thoughts and Trials

Is it sheer nonsense to use composition [Tonsatz] – or in poor German "composing" – as a teaching tool? – No, this is not quite the case. If language is a natural way and means for the expression of mankind's thoughts, the more so is music in general – and particularly the song – to express feelings and moods. We do not teach language by itself, only in combination with reading aloud or memorization of texts, poetry or prose. The main emphasis lies in enabling children to give expression to thoughts of their own and of others through stories and compositions in their own words. What is acceptable in language teaching, should also find room in the teaching of music and song. These lessons should likewise not only concentrate on memorization and sight reading, but introduce exercises in composition as well. Such exercises would not in the least be extraordinary.

In comparison to written composition, musical composition seems far more difficult to use as a teaching tool. Such an objection is not without cause, - if expectation and requirements are too high (in comparison with teaching German). For example, one would never seriously expect that schoolchildren write in metered verse, instead they write in prose. In the field of music, the "metered" form, or the heeding of complex rules of composition should also be forgone. Rather, the composition in schools should consist of "prose" (such as the various forms of recitative, up to Richard Wagner and Richard Strauss). That should allay the fears of insurmountable difficulties with composition lessons in schools. Furthermore one must not overlook that no one expects prose attempts of pupils to be published or that they should receive mention in the literary history of the future. It is only too well known, that even complete orthographic or grammatical correctness, not to mention purity of style, cannot be taught with certainty to children during school-years. Just the same: one cannot expect students to produce works equal to Beethoven's creations, and cannot declare the lack of same as a reason that composition in voice lessons is useless, just as non publication of student essays does not prove the writing of essays futile. It follows, that composition exercises make no unusual demands on a child's capability.

One cannot even call it an encumbrance. The complete omission of teaching composition is already mentioned above. (Of course, if desired, one could offer a taste of it to children in the higher grades of elementary school, in middle- and high school, just as they receive information in the theory of metrics.) As for general music education, the current curriculum suffices.

On the other hand, one need not fear that the remaining voice lesson materials will be short-changed. The new method (i.e. Eitz), in comparison to previous times, saves the threatened neglect of the memorization of songs, if such ever existed. Such danger cannot be anticipated, just as storytelling and essay writing in no way hinders the children's development of speech, likewise composition exercises will not harm knowledge and readiness in voice. The opposite is much more likely.

Now to the matter at hand! – As stated, it is natural to express moods and feelings in musical tones. Even the small child in its earliest attempts at speech will try to sing, of course not in complete arias, but completely true to the mood of the moment. It follows naturally then to start with composition in the first grade. No special preparations are necessary. In my own experience, children of various ages, including beginners, freely and without hesitation accompany poetic and prose texts, not helplessly but aesthetically quite appealing. Yet, one cannot do without structured exercises, just as they are included in the German lessons. What forms should these take? – As for myself, I tried different methods at the girl's elementary school in a 7th grade (2. school-year), and in a 5th grade (4. school-year) in 1924/25. I left teaching Easter 1925 to enter the clergy and sadly was prohibited to expand the method of these experiences; so I am limited here to report about my own exercises only in free composition. Whoever may have an interest in these may continue in this or any other way.

1. The first exercise involved finding a suitable text, from our own reader, and to sing it on a single pitch, perhaps on g. In spite of this limitation of a single pitch, enough opportunities for free self expression appropriate to the mood, with slow and fast, soft and louder singing, dividing the accented from the non-accented, i.e. the rhythm. Here I tried to learn from Eurhythmics. Here an example of the completed task:

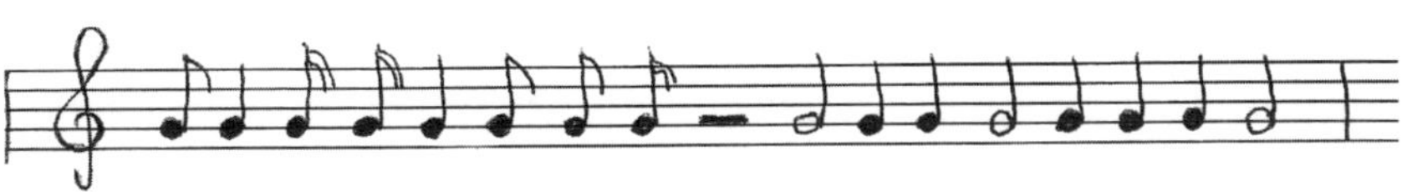

The fall-sun smiles from the sky. - Slowly and sadly leaves are falling.
[Die Herbst-sonne lacht vom Himmel - Langsam und traurig fällt das Laub]

2. Next we attempted a change in melody by moving a whole or half step from our given pitch. A whole step up

sounded bright and happy, a step down darker and serious and changed the text above in the following way:

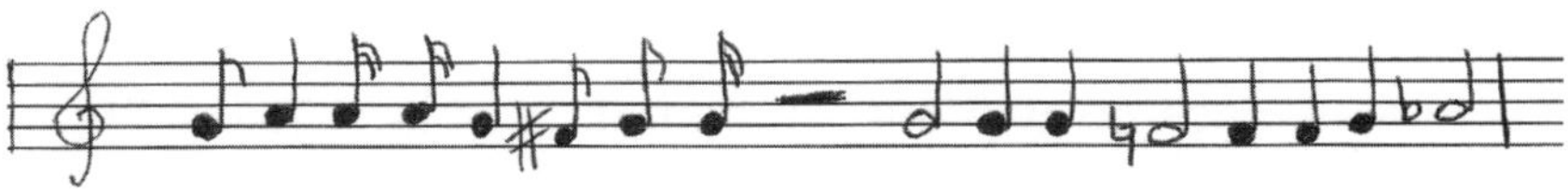

The fall-sun smiles from the sky. - Slowly and sadly leaves are falling.

3. In the last exercise we confined ourselves to moving a whole or half step at a time in one direction only. In the third exercise more freedom is granted, but still in half or whole steps at a time, in other words a scale. Upward moves on the scale expressed a lively, moving mood, while descending the scale expressed quiet and somberness. In addition, major and minor were used to strengthen these feelings. Also here an example:

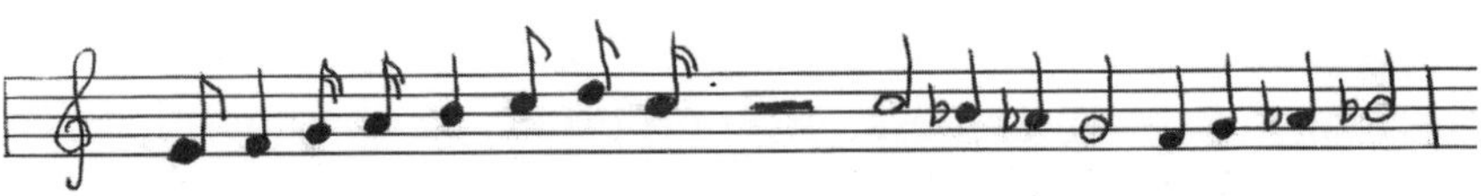

The fall-sun smiles from the sky. - Slowly and sadly leaves are falling.

4. As a fourth exercise, thirds and tonic in up and downward movements with the addition of major or minor presented many possibilities for expression as in No.3. A possible result follows:

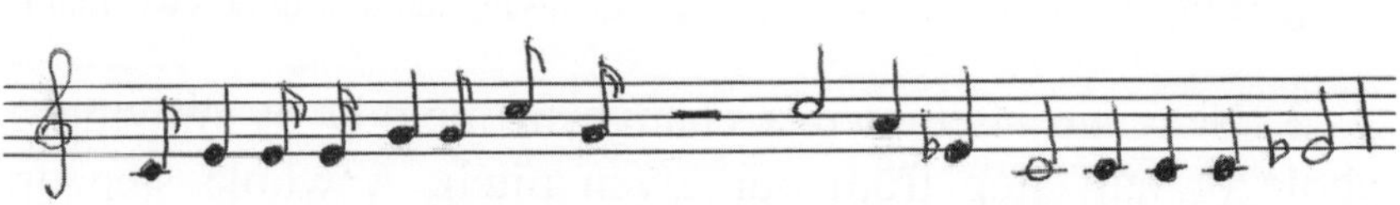

The fall-sun smiles from the sky. - Slowly and sadly leaves are falling.

Many more exercises are possible; and some were tried. We cannot explore all these here. The next step would be a suitable combination of the above. The final goal is a free musical expression of a given text.

What kind of text to choose? Our reader offers enough suitable material in prose. One can also use original texts of students and poems, of course. Just as prose can be used for composition with complex rules (Bach), so can metered speech. In the choice of text one must be mindful to not choose reading beyond the level of a child's comprehension; neither must one select material for singing, which would be inaccessible to a child's emotional state. It is also important to plan these exercises systematically and regularly, perhaps with occasional use of the reader, when German and voice are taught by the same teacher.

The possibility of accomplishing this aim is by no means associated with undue difficulties, when observing the above. Instead, time and again one is amazed how easily children adapt to the composition methods in song.

For what reason and to what purpose should the composition method be applied?

1. Do not waste, but utilize a naturally given way of expression;

2. The main reason cannot be to discover hidden talents, just as in story- telling and essay writing; however, such a possibility exists;

3. The composition method is most suitable for awakening and sharpening a sense for moods and feelings in composition and art in general;

4. It should prove most beneficial in the teaching of Richard Wagner's musical dramas and the knowledge of these is far more important than the works of third or fourth rank writers, which are currently used in schools.

5. The composition method furthers to a high degree the development of the voice, as well as the ability to recite poetry in a clear, beautiful and content-rich manner.

6. Therewith we raise the possibility of honoring the masterworks of our great poets.

7. It results in a favorable influence of one's own speech and writing styles.

The correctness of my reasoning indeed has been verified, because earlier, similar attempts were made and published in newspapers, as I belatedly found out. May the above instructions give encouragement to a similar way of teaching.

Der Tonsatz als Unterrichtsmethode. *Die Mittelschule. Zeitschrift für das gesamte mittlere Schulwesen*, 1926, 40:108-109.
– Jahr contributes to an extended discussion about didactics in teaching music in Secondary Schools; cf. other contributions on pages 265; 277; 329; 340 and 365 in 1926; most influential in these discussion was Carl Eitz „Bausteine zum Schulgesangsunterricht im Sinne der Tonsatzmethode", Leipzig: Breitkopf & Haertel 1911

LIFE SCIENCES AND THE TEACHING OF ETHICS. 1926

Old knowledge in new clothing

The modern science of life, i.e. ***biology***, does not exclusively deal with botany and zoology. It is also related to anthropology. Such a relationship is of practical value in medicine: animal experiments, blood and serum research and much more has to be mentioned, with Steinach's transplants of gonads from primates into humans perhaps the topic of the day.

Modern psychology, based on experimental psychology, also does not deal exclusively with humans any more. It uses the same methods in animal research and we have a comparative anatomic-zootomic research resulting in instructive comparisons between the human and the animal soul[*]. Indeed, even the beginning of a psychology of plants is emerging – the best known representatives are G. Th. Fechner[1] in the past and R. H. Francé[2] and Ad. Wagner[3] at present, – so that modern psychology includes all living beings in its research. Given these facts, it is only consequent when R. Eisler[4] in conclusion talks about ***Bio-Psychics*** [Bio-Psychik].

From Biopsychics it is only one step to ***Bio-Ethics*** [Bio-Ethik], i.e. to the assumption of ethical responsibilities not only towards humans but towards all living beings. In fact,

---

* Particularly recommeded among recent animal-psychological publications are Sommer, Tierpsychologie. Leipzig, and Alverdes, Tierpsychologie, Leipzig 1925.

1 G. Th. Fechner, Nanna oder das Seelenleben der Pflanzen. Leipzig 1848

2 R. H. Francé, Pflanzenpsychologie als Arbeitshypothese der Pflanzenphysiologie. Stuttgart 1909.

3 Ad. Wagner, Die Vernunft der Pflanze. Dresden 1926.

4 R. Eisler, Das Wirken der Seele. Stuttgart 1908.

bioethics is not quite a discovery of the present. Already the theologian Schleiermacher[5] calls it unethical to destroy life and formation, as they are, without a reasonable purpose, i.e. also the animal and the plant. And even earlier the poet Herder[6] requested humans to consider themselves to be in the place of other creatures in the image of the all-present feeling of the divine, to identify and to feel with each living being as much as they need it. Similarly, the philosopher Krause[7], a contemporary of Schleiermacher, requests to honor every living being as such and not destroy it without purpose. He holds that they all, plants and animals and also humans, are equal in rights, but not identical in rights, each according to the necessary requirement to reach their destination.

As far as animals are concerned, such an ethical obligation has become self-evident for some time now, at least in the form of not making them suffer needlessly[8]. As an especially attractive role model from the past we may, particularly in this year, recall Francesco of Assisi and his great love for animals in our memories. – With plants it is different: it may be contrary to some people to consider certain ethical obligations towards plants. But this is not so. Already Paul in his poetic reference to the yearning hope[9] of all creatures (i.e. also animals and plants) awakens our compassion with them. – A comparison piece would be in the third act of Richard Wagner's "Parsifal" with its moving atmospheric statements: In pious devotion, humans at least on Good Friday respect stalks

---

[5] Schleiermacher, Philosophische Sittenlehre (Kirchmann) 1870.

[6] Herder, Ideen zur Philosophie der Geschichte der Menschheit. Riga und Leipzig 1785.

[7] K. Chr. Fr. Krause, Das System der Rechtsphilosophie. (Röder) Leipzig 1874.

[8] The best publication in this area still is J. Bregenzer. Tierethik. Bamberg 1894.

[9] Römerbrief Kap. 8;19-22. Recently J. Martius published „Die Unsterblichkeit der Pflanze", Stuttgart 1838.

and flowers by walking carefully in the meadows in order not to hurt them. – In this context we also should mention the fairy tale by Anderson about the angel, who did not carry only the soul of the child, which prematurely died, into heaven but also a number of flowers, including a dried-out wild flower which had been his greatest and only pleasure when he was alive, a fatally ill child of poor parents in a dim basement. And God held all flowers close to his heart; but the poor dried-out wild flower he kissed, and she got voices and song from angels floating around God. – While these are only examples of poetic vision, it may be true what Richard Wagner had Hans Sachs say

> "All creative writing and poetry
> Are nothing but *true* interpretation of dreams
> [*Wahr*traumdeuterei]".

We recognize this, when we familiarize ourselves with the serious plant-ethics concepts of a matter-of-fact philosopher, such as Ed. von Hartmann[10], who died only twenty years ago. In an article on flower-luxury he writes about a cut flower: "She is an organism deadly hurt, but only her colors not yet destroyed, a head still there, but separated from the torso. – – Whenever I see a rose in a glass of water or tied into a bouquet, I cannot fight the unpleasant thought that a human being has murdered a flower life for the sole purpose to enjoy his/her eyes, heartless enough to not sense the unnatural death under the appearance of life. – – And if I see a masterpiece of a flower arrangement, a big basket overflowing with most precious wire-strung blossoms, I feel pressed to admire a la-

[10] Psychological aspects are discussed by W. v. Schnehen. E. v. Hartmann und die Planzenpsychologie. Stuttgart 1908.

dies headdress of many pierced butterflies, broken on the wheel and still struggling"[11]. The plant-ethics obligations associated with such a view are clear, of course.

The realization of such ethical obligations towards all living beings seems utopian. But we should not neglect that ethical obligations towards living beings in practicality are related to their "necessity" (Herder) or their "destination" (Krause). Now, the requirements of animals are much less complex in number and content than those of humans. This is even more true for the plant, so that ethical obligations towards plants – which already (if not in general, but in practice) are smaller than towards animals – are less difficult. Also, the principle of struggle for life is important, – a principle which in some way even modifies our ethical obligations towards humans. Within these parameters there remain always many opportunities for bioethical activity. An introduction on how this can be achieved in the fields of animal ethics is exemplified by various paragraphs of animal protection in the penal codes of different civilized countries[12]. In the fields of plant ethics our compassion leads the way and hinders us from decapitating plants right and left with a walking stick when being on a stroll outside or from picking flowers and throwing them away without respect after a while; similarly we abhor the blind rage of destruction by unrefined lads breaking the stems of young trees along the road. – This results in the guiding principle for our actions in ***the Bio-ethical Imperative:***

[11] Ed. von Hartmann. Der Blumenluxus. 1885.

[12] These materials are collected and discussed by R. v. Hippel. Die Tierquälerei in der Strafgesetzgebung des In- und Auslandes. Berlin 1891. For additional practical recommendations see Kyber: Tierschutz und Kultur, Stuttgart and Heilbronn 1925.

"Respect every living being in general as an end in itself and treat it, if possible, as such!"

As far as classroom teaching is concerned, it becomes possible to also influence the character [Gesinnung] in scientific disciplines educationally. Thus, these disciplines in some way become character formation disciplines as well. This is of great importance in regard to a timely request for environmental protection [Naturschutz]. We don't need to support environment protection only from an aesthetic point of view, rather from pointing out that it is horrible to torture animals, to senselessly destroy plants, and to deface God's free nature by thrown away paper, egg shells, or broken glass, – thus it will be elevated to a serious obligation in ethics.

Wissenschaft vom Leben und Sittenlehre. *Die Mittelschule. Zeitschrift für das gesamte mittlere Schulwesen*, 1926, 40:604-605 [15. Dezember 1926]

BIO-ETHICS. 1927

Reviewing the ethical relations of humans towards animals and plants

The strict distinction between animal and human being [Mensch], prevalent in our European culture until the end of the 18th century, cannot be supported anymore. The European soul wrestled until the French Revolution for a unity of religious, philosophical, and scientific knowledge; but such a unity had to be abandoned under the pressure of more information.

It will always be the credit of modern natural sciences to finally render an unbiased study of the world [Weltgeschehen]. We would not be seekers of truth today, if we had given up the results of animal experimentation, blood research etc... On the other hand, we cannot deny that precisely these scientific triumphs of the human spirit have infringed upon the dominant position of the human being in the world in general. Philosophy, formerly guiding ideas [Leitgedanken] for the natural sciences, now has to build her systems following the specific knowledge of the natural sciences, – and it was only a poetic-philosophical [dichterphilosophische] interpretation of Darwin's insight, when Nietzsche considered humans to be a somewhat inferior stage towards a higher stage in evolution, as a "rope extended between animal and superman [Übermensch]."

What follows from this turmoil? First: the fundamental equation of humans and animals as objects in psychology. Today, it [psychology] does not restrict itself to human beings, but applies the same methods to animals as well; and, as documented by comparative anatomical-zoological research, quite instructive comparisons between human soul and animal soul have been done. Yes, even beginnings of plant psychology are visible; – the most prominent representatives are G. Th. Fechner in the past, R. H. Francé, Ad. Wagner and the Indian Bose at present, so that modern research in psychology covers all living beings in research. Given these circumstances, it is only logical when R. Eisler speaks of *Bio-Psychics* [Bio-Psychik] (science of the soul of all that lives).

From Bio-Psychics it is only a step to *Bio-Ethics*, i.e. the assumption of moral obligations not only towards humans, but towards all forms of life. In reality, bio-ethics is not just a discovery of modern times. An especially attractive example from the past is the figure of St. Francis of Assisi (1182-1226) with his great love towards animals, his warm sympathy for all forms of life, centuries before Rousseau's romanticism for the entire nature.

When the unity of the European weltanschauung eroded at the end of the Baroque period, European intellectual life for the first time was receptive towards the influence of foreign worlds of thought [Gedankenwelten] without prejudice. Already Herder's comprehensive spirit – probably the most sensitive in those days for things to come – expected of humans, based on the image of an all encompassing deity, that they project themselves into each and every creature and sense with it the way it needs. Such a reasoning already reminds us of the Indian philosophy, which by the way of England just had been discovered. But only during the time of Romanticism has India really influenced European intellectual life, including Germany, its most important province at that time. The teaching of reincarnation, as developed in India, has influenced the reasoning of Indian schools of philosophy, especially the school of Sankya. An offspring of this school is yoga teaching, drawing the most rigorous consequences from those thought processes. The yoga repentant [Jogabüßer] under no circumstances is allowed to live at the cost of co-creatures; above all, he shall under no circumstances kill any animal, and only under certain settings enjoy vegetable foods. He has to wear a veil over his mouth in order not to inhale even a small living being; for the same reason he has to filter drinking water and shall not take a bath. The passion to not harm a living being in the process of self-preservation even leads some Indian repentant to eat horse manure. If in this context Buddha is mentioned, one has to stress that especially this religious leader refused such fanatic self-harm of the yoga preachers. Buddha forbade, that food be based on animal products, but fully allows vegetable based foods.

How thoroughly Buddha himself and his teachings believe in reincarnation [Seelenwanderung] is very well demonstrated to us Europeans in the Jatakas stories, beautiful Buddhist tales he himself told of his former life. He not only claims that he has lived as a human being before, but also remembers his former lives as an elephant, a gazelle, a crab etc... Even more beautiful than in Francis of Assisi, these narratives express the thought, that a human being is in essence related to all creatures.

Such sequences of reasoning caused similar thoughts in European intellectual life, even if not in such a strict version. Theologian Schleiermacher (1768-1834) declared it to be immoral to destroy life and formation [Leben und Gestaltung], as they are, if there is no reasonable cause to do so. Similarly, the philosopher Krause, a contemporary of Schleiermacher, requests to respect each and every living being and not to destroy it without reason. Because, they all, plants and animals, also humans, have Similar Rights, but not Equal Rights, depending on the requirements for reaching their specific destiny. The philosopher Schopenhauer, who claimed as special importance of his ethics as based primarily on the sentiment of compassion, required towards animals as well, openly referred to the Indian intellectual world [Gedankenwelt]. Via Richard Wagner, who was strongly influenced by Schopenhauer and a compassionate animal lover and friend of animal protection, those thoughts have become a common value for a broadest group of people.

Thus, regarding animals such a rule has become evident, at least as far as needless torture is concerned. With plants it is different, so. For some, it seems at first unreasonable to have certain ethical obligations towards plants. But already [Apostle] Paul directed our compassion towards animals and plants. Comparable are the illuminated sentimental [verklärt stimungsvollen] interpretations in Richard Wagner's 3rd act of "Parsifal". In pious devotion, humans at least on Good Friday avoid hurting stalks and flowers in the fields by walking more carefully. But also in the thoughts of plant ethics by a sober philosopher such as Eduard von Hartmann, who passed away 20 years ago, we find similar thoughts. In an article on flower-luxury he describes a cut flower: "She is an organism deadly hurt, but only her colors not yet destroyed, a head still there, but separated from the torso. – Whenever I see a rose in a glass of water or strung on a wire in a bouquet, I cannot fight the unpleasant thought that a human being has murdered a flower life for the sole purpose to enjoy his/her eyes while dying, eyes heartless enough, not to sense an unnatural death under the appearance of life."

A majority of people naturally is not as sensitive as Ed. von Hartmann. However, everyone knows quite well, that plants are living beings, and cutting flowers hurts; but the thought that the flower could sense it, is distant. The concept of a plant-soul so far has not taken hold in us. Additionally, we know that flowers also die and dry out, while they are on the plant, and therefore one does not take issue with cutting flowers, in particular when they were cultivated for that specific purpose.

Thus, we start from a totally different point of view than the Indian fanatics, who do not want to hurt any living entity. Also, our regulations by law and police protect specific plants and flowers in certain areas (such as plants in the Alps) are based on totally different assumptions. The police state [Polizeistaat] intends to protect those plants from becoming extinct in those areas, also to be enjoyed by other people in the future. Whenever plants are abundant, the state does not intervene to protect them as an end in themselves.

Also, our concept of animal protection rests on a decidedly different foundation than the attitude of the Indians. When we read in the novel "Holy Hate" [Der heilige Haß] by Richard Voß, that a Rodya-boy, i.e. a member of a despised caste, does even not want to kill a snake, because "also the snakes are our brothers and sisters", we do not accept such a reasoning; we actually hold it to be our duty to kill harmful animals, if we can. We have our farm animals killed by the butcher and the harmless prey by the hunter, because we want to eat meat, which in our areas some feel they cannot do without, while in tropical countries vegetarian food is abundantly available. Our animal protection, thus, has a utilitarian aspect, which is boldly disregarded by the Indians, while we content ourselves with avoidance of unnecessary suffering. Unfortunately, legal regulations against prevention or punishment of those cruelties are not strong enough in all civilized countries [Kulturländern] yet. But, we are on the road of progress and animal protection gets more and more support in wider circles, so that no decent human being [anständiger Mensch] will accept without criticism, that a thoughtless lout [Flegel] without any thought beheads flowers with a stick when on a hike or that children break flowers only to throw them away after a few steps. Our self-education, in this regard, already has made considerable progress, but we have to go further, so that the guiding rule for our actions may be the bio-ethical demand:

"Respect every living being on principle as an end in itself and treat it, if possible, as such!"

Bio-Ethik. Eine Umschau über die ethischen Beziehungen des Menschen zu Tier und Pflanze. *Kosmos. Handweiser für Naturfreunde* 1927, 24(1): 2-4

DEATH AND THE ANIMALS, 1928

Contemplating the 5th Commandment

"Thou shalt not kill", thus are we Christians warned by the 5th commandment. – Does not killing always relate to something alive? Since the commandment does not expressly forbid the killing of humans only, should we therefore not also apply it to other living beings, especially the animals? Perhaps the artist-painter Fidus was right on target with his painting of "You shall not kill" [Du sollst nicht töten]: a child, reflecting innocence and purity, spreads its own protective arms in front of a deer to save it from the hunter's deadly bullet!?

Are animals so close to us that we should acknowledge and treat them as our "neighbors"? – No doubt, considerable differences do exist between man and the animals, and modern sciences acknowledge this. However, that does not prevent biology and the life-sciences to utilize related trends in practical application, especially since many of these trends had also been acknowledged by Darwin. To mention here: animal experiments, blood testing, blood-protein research, transplants of animal tissue to man, as well as others. On a spiritual plain, interesting parallels between man and animal have emerged as well, so that both share not only physiologic but also psychological "nearness".

We should not find this disquieting; to the contrary, we should be proud that the discoveries of adventurous human spirits in recent times already are contained in the core of the Holy Scriptures. Genesis, the 1st book of Moses, speaks of a "soul" of animals (Gen. 9:16). The Preacher Salomon also presupposes a soul in them, similar to humans and asks doubtfully:

> "Who knows, whether the spirit of man goes upward, and the spirit of the beast goes down into the earth?" (Ec. 3:21)

In any case, all creatures, be it man or beast, long for delivery from death and transiency, as taught by the apostle Paul in the epistle to the Roman congregation (Romans 8:18-23), a sign, that already of old a commonality between man and animal was recognized. Small wonder, that later on Franz von Assisi called all living creatures his sisters and brothers, and that Herder, too, saw in animals "man's older brothers". If that be so, one can grasp that when God made the covenant with humankind, he did likewise with the animals, as written in the 1st book of Moses (Genesis 9:9-10. 17), and in Hosea (Hos 2:18-20). Even in the kingdom to come there will be a place for them, as written in Isaiah:

> "Wolves shall dwell with lambs,
> and the leopard shall lie with the young goat,
> and the calf and the lion and the fattened calf together;
> and a little child shall lead them.
> The cow and the bear shall graze;
> their young shall lie together;
> and the lion shall eat straw like the ox.
> The nursing child shall play over the hole of the cobra,
> and the weaned child shall put his hand on the adder's den." (Isa. 11:6-8)

In his table-talks no one lesser than Luther himself shared the belief of an acceptance of animals in the kingdom to come.

Given that the natural sciences as well as the Holy Scriptures hold animals in such high regard, it follows that we Christians have ethical obligations to them. We should indeed apply the 5th commandment to animals. Schleiermacher, most noted theologian of the newer times, expressly considered it immoral to destroy life and formation wherever established, including animals, without reasonable cause.

However, the fulfillment of the 5th commandment extended to animals seems utopian: Slaughter and killing of animals is hardly avoidable, even if done only for needed supply of a growing population. The struggle for life [Kampf ums Dasein] makes this a necessity. However much we may regret it, this same principle also influences our ethical behaviors towards our fellow man. In our entire life and activities, be it in politics, in economics, in the office, in the workshop, in the fields, the basic goals are in no way primarily directed by love, but rather by struggle with some kind of competitors of ours. Mostly we are not quite aware of this, as long as the struggle does not breach the limits of the law. In such struggle for life we humans deliberately and consciously use human power, human health, human life, not only in times of war, but also in 'peaceful' life such as in cultural development, especially in some of the industries. In spite of all this no one considers the 5th commandment a utopian charge. As our attitude towards animals – as determined by struggle for life – basically does not fall outside our attitude towards man, the commandment can and must be valid here as well, an ideal and a point of reference for our moral strife.

But what effect will this ideal have in reality, given the mentioned restrictions in sparing the lives of animals? – Schleiermacher requests to kill animals only then, when a reasonable cause demands it. Besides, animal protection laws and societies give us further guidelines on how to be "merciful to our beasts".

The admonition to spare animal-life is absolutely valid, without any regard to being to our advantage, as ethics in general does not and may not ask those questions. Richard Wagner, as does Schopenhauer, stresses this point especially: "Everyone, who at the sight of a tortured animal suffers outrage, is so moved singly by compassion; and whoever unites with others for the protection of animals is solely motivated by compassion, i.e. empathy by nature indifferent and inconsiderate of any calculated gain."

In view of this principle it is interesting and useful to raise the following question: "What effects will this expansion of our ethical duties beyond man to animals have on our relationship to our fellow man? Should we fear that the attention to the needs of our fellow man could be diminished because of our obligation to the animals?" – Exactly the opposite occurs: When we nurture in our breast a feeling heart toward the animals, we will not withhold compassion and help from suffering humankind. He, who has love so great that it reaches beyond the human-only realm and can see holiness in the poorest creature, he will also see and highly regard the divine in his poorest and lowest brothers, he will not limit himself to a certain societal class, interest group, or certain party. On the other hand, cruelty to animals is a sign of an unrefined character, which could also be dangerous to the human environment. Many great thinkers attest to this fact and the philosopher Kant also states that the compassionate and merciful dealings with animals are a duty man owes to himself.

Above all, the sparing of animal life as far as possible is a duty to God; if we want to honor the creator, we must regard with awe and respect his creatures, the animals as well, the more that we know he loves them too (Jon. 4:11) and bore them in mind as he commanded:

"Thou shalt not kill!"

Der Tod und die Tiere. Eine Betrachtung über das 5. Gebot, *Mut und Kraft*, Halle 1928, 5(1): 5-6

ANIMAL PROTECTION AND ETHICS. 1928

Compassion with animals shows up as an empirically given phenomenon of the human soul. This fact has been voiced, among others, by the poet and philosopher Herder in his "Ideas in History of Humankind" [Ideen zur Geschichte der Menschheit]. The fact, that this phenomenon is more or less present in a normal human soul, is also assumed by the German Penal Code when expressing in paragraph 360 (13) that cruelty to animals is a public offense. Exceptions, which of course are there, cannot change the truth of such a psychological observation, similarly as the existence of blind people can be used to argue that the capability of seeing is not an essential part of humans. Such compassion now is the central motive of the idea of animal protection [Tierschutz]. Thus, it does not calculate whether or not one has any benefit from it; e.g. Richard Wagner in an open letter to Ernst von Weber, under the influence of Schopenhauer's "On the Foundation of Morality" [Über das Fundament der Moral], argues: "Everyone, who reacts indignant when witnessing the suffering of an animal, is motivated solely by compassion, and who works together with others in protecting animals does so similarly only out of compassion, naturally not of calculations of utility by an otherwise unconcerned and determined compassion."

And if someone does not accept the unconditional nature of Animal Ethics (as one may call it, following Bregenzer, who was the first to publish a scientific Animal Ethics [Tierethik] from an ethical-legal position), one nevertheless may not suppress the question of the relationship between animal protection and ethics, respectively seek to answer such a question. In other words: what are the consequences in our relationships towards our fellow humans when we extend our moral obligations beyond humans towards animals? Don't we have to fear, that we will turn away our awareness from the misery of the latter towards the first? The philosopher Eduard von Hartmann, who, by the way, is not hostile against animals, voices those concerns in his article "Our Relationship towards Animals" [Unsere Stellung zu den Tieren]. He gives the example of a "dry old maid", feeding meats and sweets to her pug while letting her employees go hungry. He also finds love towards animals among embittered misanthropes, cold and cruel judges of heretics and bloodthirsty heroes of revolutions. While these cases are true, Hartmann's arguments only target *false* animal love. This kind of false love also may be used towards humans. It is expressed in disgusting pampering, in unjustifiable preferences, in cronyism [Vetternwirtschaft], and unfortunately widely spread otherwise. But if such false love of people is not a valid argument against ethics, so is occasionally occurring false love of animals no demonstration against the justification of animal protection.

This is the issue: When we have a compassionate heart towards animals, then we will not withhold our compassion and help towards suffering humans. If someone's love is great enough to go beyond the borders of human-only and sees the sanctity even in the most miserable creature, he or she will find this sanctity as well in the poorest and lowest fellow human, will hold it high and will not reduce it to class or society, interest group, one party or what else may be considered. On the other hand, senseless cruelty towards animals is an indication of an unrefined character and is dangerous towards the human environment as well. Among other thinkers, philosopher Kant expressively has hinted at this fact of highest importance for social ethics, when in "Metaphysische Anfangsgründe der Tugendlehre" he calls the careful and compassionate treatment of animals a human obligation towards oneself. The word from Count Leo Tolstoy: "From killing animals to killing humans, it is only one step" might be overly strong; but his position expresses Kant's concept and understanding. This is also the case for R. von Hippel, a jurist, who has collected and organized most of the relevant historical and statistical materials.

But effective and successful animal protection is only possible, when enough knowledge and at least some understanding of nature are present. The reason is that we only can protect animals in reality, when we are somewhat knowledgeable about their physiological and psychological properties and life conditions. Therefore one of the main goals of the animal protection movement is the promotion of such a kind of knowledge and a better understanding of nature, – awakening, broadening, and deepening it. Such an interest in nature will by itself not limit itself to animals, but on the other side also towards plants and (what is most important in this content) towards humans as well. If such a goal will only be reached in part, then we can, for sure, expect a positive influence on humans and their way of life, i.e. in the attitude of a normal and healthy naturalness, which has nothing to do with a limitless life of over-excited, unhealthy, and thereby unnatural urges, which quite often wrongly are considered to be natural. The fact that the promotion of knowledge and understanding of nature and of a true love for nature will also have a positive effect on sexual ethics does not need to be demonstrated additionally.

If, indeed, it is true that a correctly understood and executed animal protection works positively on ethics, then it is also true that it has a value in public education and public knowledge; and this may not be underrated at all. On the other hand, everyone, who is active in animal protection, will support as much as possible general ethical activities, which, as already mentioned, cannot ignore or be silent about animal ethics, because this is also indirectly supportive of animal protection.

The fact of a close interrelationship between animal protection and ethics finally is based on the reality that we not only have moral obligations to fellow humans, but also to animals, even to plants – in short: to all forms of life – , so that we can speak about "Bio-Ethics".

As such, Bio-Ethics is not just an idea of modern times. – Already Montaigne, a skeptic, was the first Frenchman – so far being the first representative of a modern ethos of sentiment – who dared to reason, that all living beings have entitlement of being treated based on ethical principles: we owe justice towards humans, mildness and compassion towards all other creatures who will have a benefit from it. So he wrote in his "Essays" in 1588. – Precisely in the same sense, Herder expects from humans to follow the example of a God, who transfigures with sentiment every living entity and is empathetic with it as much as it can feel and need. He explicitly includes plants in this. – Highlights are reached by the theologian Schleiermacher and philosopher K. Chr. F. Krause. The first one, in his "Philosophische Ethik", declares it to be immoral to destroy life and forms of life, wherever they are, i.e. including animals and plants, without a reasonable cause associated with such an act. The latter, a contemporary of Schleiermacher, requests in his "Rechtsphilosophie" that every living being be treasured as such and not be destroyed without reason: because they all, plants and animals, also humans, are of equal standing [gleichberechtigt]. But they are not identical, and each only in a way which is a necessary requirement to reach its destination, as we read in Krause's "Abriss der Philosophie des Rechts". – A note in the diary of the poet Hebbel reminds us of the intuition of Herder, according to which not only humans, but everything living and moving [was lebt und webt] sees an inscrutable divine light, which one can access only via love.

It must be mentioned in this context that one has tried and still is trying – the longer the more – to support the bioethical thought by biological and biopsychological arguments, and not without success.

At first hand, it might appear utopian to realize such moral obligations towards all living entities. But we can not overlook that such moral obligations towards a living entity in reality are determined by its "needs" [Bedürfnisse] (Herder), respectively its "destiny" (Krause). So, the needs of animals seem to be lower in quantity and less complicated in content than those of humans. This is even more true for plants, so that practical moral obligations, which are already there towards animals (if not basically, but practically), create less difficulties. Additionally we have to take into account the principle of struggle for life and existence, a principle which in some way also modifies our obligations towards fellow humans, even if we might feel unhappy about it. Our entire life and activity in politics, in business, in administration, in the laboratory, in the workshop, in the fields is – as Naumann has underlined – in its reasoning and goals not focusing on love in the first place, quite often rather focused on struggle with some sort of fellow competitors. Quite often we don't recognize it, as long as such a struggle is without hate and in an open and legally accepted way. As much as we cannot avoid the struggle with fellow humans, similarly the struggle for survival [Kampf ums Dasein] with other living entities is unavoidable. Nevertheless, neither in the first nor in the second case, we will lose the idea of moral obligations as a principle. The paragraphs of animal protection laws in the penal codes of civilized countries and the activities of animal protection societies give testimony, in which ways animal protection becomes practical. In the field of plant ethics, our intuition will hinder us from killing plants right and left with a cane during a stroll, or from picking flowers only in order to throw them away after a short while, or when we detest the blind acts of destruction by ruffian lads breaking the crowns of young trees along the road or in the woods.

From all this follows as guidance for our moral acts the *Bio-ethical Imperative:*

Respect every living being, including animals, as an end in itself, and treat it, if possible, as such! And if someone does not accept the validity of this principle, as far as it is concerned with animals and plants, then, in repeating what already was said, one nevertheless should follow it in recognition of the moral obligation toward human society in general.

Tierschutz und Ethik in ihren Beziehungen zueinander. *Ethik. Sexual- und Gesellschaftsethik. Organ des Ethikbundes,* 1928, 4(6/7): 100-102

SOCIAL AND SEXUAL ETHICS IN THE DAILY PRESS. 1928

Thoughts occasioned by "Pressa"

All ethical reflections find a real purpose only when work is done, either theoretical or practical. Even as *practical* confirmation is most important – especially by role model – nevertheless *theoretical* enlightening information [Aufklärung] by word and text should not be underestimated. – Regarding the spoken word, i.e. the form of private influence from person to person, is concerned, also lectures and presentations, the success by means of speaking and talking should not be overestimated, in particular since these lectures sometimes do not draw too many people. Radio probably has a much greater influence.

This leads to the printed word as far as theoretical enlightening information is concerned.

Here, we have to mention in the first place

the professional press.

The professional press has the great advantage that its opens its pages exclusively to issues of controversial ethical problems, being basically more or less independent from those people, who are neutral or even hostile to these concerns. But a certain deficiency is connected with such an advantage: The professional journal reaches only those, who already are members of such a movement or otherwise close to it. Therefore, an immediate influence on the masses is missing. – Such a deficiency is even greater as far as books are concerned; on one side the purchase price is deterring, on the other side, not everyone has time and leisure to read a not so easily digested and sometimes quite voluminous publication. Additionally, the book market is not short of publication on ethical issues, so it is difficult to make the right selection.

Thus, the most important issue is still to review

the daily press

in regard to its importance for ethics. From the point of view of the "Ethikbund", newspapers are not without deficiencies. The daily press by far has not the same space available as a professional journal or even a book. Also, the daily press sometimes has to be careful to handle certain issues in recognition of its sponsors, parties, advertiser or subscribers. – This deficiency however is balanced with great advantages. First and most importantly, there is wide distribution of the daily press. Immense amounts of paper are used daily to produce newspapers. Millions of eyes review on a daily basis the multimillion lines of newspapers. Not even the most widely read professional journal nor book can compete with that. Such an incredible distribution is matched with a similarly incredible influence, whatever else one thinks about the usefulness of newspapers. Events going on in the city, in the county, in the fatherland, activities in the wide world, – where do we get information about those if not in the daily press? It also analyses the big political and economical issues and events, – things we need to know in order to recognize and to fulfill our social obligations; – we also get information about food prices, how to dress, what the costs of certain garments are, and products recommendable, which is not in direct but in indirect relationship to ethics. And as the newspaper knows, men don't live by bread and other daily stuff alone; it reports about intellectual and spiritual issues as well, and so ethics cannot be missed.

Finally: as newspapers will only off and on bring articles of ethical content, not too long and preferably in a feuilleton style, the creation of interest and understanding among lay readers – also from this perspective the importance of the daily press for ethics, including social ethics and sexual ethics – should not be underestimated.

Thus, the relationship between newspapers and ethics must be strongly emphasized and in any case. This is independently from being a supporter or enemy of the daily press. Also irrelevant is whether one considers the press to be an expression of public opinion or rather being the "producer" or modifier of such a public opinion in the first place. – The newspaper friend will use it as an instrument of ethical work, in particular because in this way he will not only have an opportunity to express ethical reasoning but also to distribute it widely. – But even the sworn enemy of the newspaper will not refrain from at least working *with* or supporting it, even if only for the purpose (if this is justifiable or not, is irrelevant in this regard) to influence it positively. The *possibility* of such an influence is always given, if one recognizes the newspaper as an expression of public opinion. And if one considers the pages in the newspaper to be a medium to establish or at least strongly influence public opinion, then from an ethical point of view, it becomes even an *obligation*, to take part in this type of character formation [Gesinnungsbildung], actively and with good knowledge and conscience.

To start with the most suitable newspapers is a matter of pragmatism. Also important are close contacts with correspondents. Best advice can be sought from experts in both areas: ethics and newspaper expertise. To use this opportunity is of particular importance for the good cause, to which social ethics and sexual ethics definitely belong, and is highly recommended.

Soziale und sexuelle Ethik in der Tageszeitung. *Ethik. Sexual- und Gesellschaftsethik. Organ des Ethikbundes,* 1928, 4(10/11): 149-150.
– Jahr's thoughts were occasioned by the International Press Exhibit, in short „Pressa", which Oberbuergermeister Konrad Adenauer opened in May 1928 and therewith established Koeln's reputation as a convention center.

WAYS TO SEXUAL ETHICS. 1928

The sexual problem is one of the hottest problems in present-day ethics. One should not miss, that in olden days, yes, even in ancient times the same topic had surfaced among the most different peoples. Only, it was not given the broad latitude as in younger days, especially our present.

As a means, perhaps the only means, to stave off and prevent sexual-ethics harm to youth as well as adults, since the 18th century until today, was adequate rational information [Aufklärung] about sex life and its physiological base. For example, Rousseau, whose 150th anniversary of death we celebrate this year on the 2nd of July, in his 4th book of the education novel "Emile, ou de l'education" advocates reasonable sexual information for young people above the age of sixteen. Rousseau regards it such an essential part of reasoned enlightenment, that he even planned visits for his imagined pupil Emil with syphilis patients and brothels, all for clearness' sake. As a significant friend and advocate of Rousseau's ideas, Basedow, a contemporary and acquaintance of Goethe, gained notoriety in Germany. He likewise advocated sex education, as did many youth-educators with and after him. In these circles the suggestion originated to demonstrate suitable cadaver resections for better visualization of sex education. We see clearly that reasoned teaching on sexual matters is just as valuable today as in the "times of Enlightment" [Aufklärungszeit], as Kant calls it. Numerous lectures, exhibits, films, writings and sundries attest to this (some among them worthless and even harmful).

How to judge this diffuse rationality-oriented attitude towards issues in sexual ethics? – Without doubt, thought and rationality can and must be applied to all matters, including ethical as well as sexual ethics, nay – it is necessary. To deny this necessity also means to deny the pursuit of the problem in question, as well as any progress, which might result from it. Above all, that would be the worst possible mistake. In Goethe's "Faust" Mephistopheles rightfully says:

> If you despise rationality and knowledge,
> the highest power of a human
> – – – – – – – –
> then I already have caught you, for sure!

So far, all should be clear. Only, we may not overlook that man is not exclusively a thinking being, rationality is not representative of all the other impulses of the mind. The omission of this long established psychological fact is widespread and it is often forgotten that man is endowed with strong drives and sentiments. And because of the strength of these inner drives, it is extremely difficult to subordinate sexual ethics to rationality alone: we have to recognize that the sexual drive may be especially powerful. In general, these drives are so strong, that man commonly gives in to them, even if reason tells him that he will be harmed. As an example of the real drive for self-preservation: a drowning man will grasp the last straw, as the proverb says, or, also his savior, if there is one, even though he knows it will complicate his rescue, might even make it impossible. The drive for self-preservation works blindly in this case and reason has no power to sway. A similarly impelling force of resistance exists in sex drive, especially if strongly endowed or deranged through illness. To regard the last extreme case: A homosexually oriented male in his soul might regard his sexual orientation as wrong, unnatural, or ill; so for the remainder of his life he is unhappy. Even though his rationality might regard this as abnormal, he cannot alter that drive. Often he cannot even totally suppress acting on it. Similarly, this also applies to both sexes concerning simple or mutual masturbation, a widespread bad custom. Even the natural, more or less healthy sex-drive will often triumph over reason and teachings. (It goes without saying that a phlegmatic person is in less danger than a sanguine person.) In such a situation it is evident that on occasion well-meant rational teachings can have the opposite of the intended results, especially in individuals who can easily be aroused. – An example of old is found in the Bible: Even though matters of the sex life are easily and freely discussed, any enticing details are missing. Double meanings and sultry atmospheres are absent. Yet until the present day, lecturing to youth from such passages is considered dangerous. And similarly today, we find illustration of this with public educational films: While regular educational films are poorly attended; sex education films are always well attended. This, without a doubt, puts into question that the interest is purely that of reason, but much more – if not always consciously – it is prompted by sex drive.

It is nothing new, that rationality alone is not the only momentum driving the demands of promotion of sex ethics. Formerly mentioned Rousseau and Basedow are outspoken opponents of this exaggerated "reasonable-ing" [Vernünfteelns]. Already in yonder times attempts were made to directly influence, from childhood on, the so-called "moral feeling" [moralisches Gefühl] in sex ethics. Of course, this was aimed at the furthering of sex ethics in adults. – However, focusing on practical issues and effects, let's consider the following. – What practical consequences would result from the significant impact of human drives and their influence and impact on sex ethics? It is self-evident, to explicitly repeat the already stated, that one cannot do without rational sex education. It is only our reason that can convince us to consider seriously not only the rational aspect, but the physiological and, in the most modern sense, especially the psychological aspect as well. – One of the means to this is to care for active religiosity. – Much is expected of the awakening and strengthening of "moral sentiments" [moralische Gefühle], as they were called during the time of enlightenment; in our specific field it would entail a cultivation of a sense of shame. – To accomplish this, it is essential to remove damaging influences. We must keep a keen eye on the widely offered, mostly illustrated literature on sexual topics. This attention must not only be directed towards new publications, but include classical writings. I only want to mention here the (unedited) Tales of a "1001 Nights", "Decamerone" by Boccaccio and "The Adventures of Casanova". That these writings were not isolated in the past is proven by the repeated serious warnings of already mentioned pedagogue Basedow against those unsuitable, sensually arousing readings. Most important would be a purposeful lifestyle. Included in this is a balanced diet with properly sized portions at timely intervals, hygienic principles applied to clothing, living quarters (especially sleeping arrangements), that work and recreation are in due proportions to each other (not too much or too little of either), and that instead of social and worldly pleasures, there should be physical exercise and enjoyment in an ever more neglected nature (sports, hiking, gardening, etc.). Guard the Golden Rule of: Early to bed and early to rise! A further address of important issues (for example the question of alcohol) cannot be made here at this time. Those are best addressed by a competent and experienced physician.

Of special importance in childhood and youth is a direct influence in sex ethics, not accessed from rational education alone; for one must always balance the danger of moral harm against the possibility of a successful impact in education. Here starts the development of sex ethics in the soon to be adult, no proof needed.

Wege zum sexualen Ethos. *Ethik. Sexual- und Gesellschaftsethik. Organ des Ethikbundes,* 1928, 4(10/11): 161-163

TWO BASIC MORAL PROBLEMS: OPPOSITION AND ALLIANCE IN SOCIAL LIFE. 1929

[EGOISM AND ALTRUISM]

There are two highly important basic issues in individual ethics and social ethics:

(I) the egoistic or egocentric, and

(II) the altruistic position, also called the sense for justice, compassion, pity, love (not in the sexual sense) etc.

Philosophical and theological academic ethics do not always use these parallel terms in similar ways. It may be allowed for reasons of simplicity to use "egoistic" respective "egocentric" as a psychological fact, the result of which is the struggle for life, and "altruism", "love", etc. representing the opposite attitude of feeling, willing, and reasoning, connected with appropriate practical consequences.

I.

First, to the egocentric attitude, i.e. the interest in me myself: We should not neglect that such an attitude originally is an intuitive, instinctive drive. Only secondarily, if at all, it becomes a conscientious reasoning form of thinking in regard to a potentially justified struggle-for-life attitude and the best methods in such a struggle. – We recognize already the struggle for life among plants, by means of abundant multiplication, unpleasant odor or taste, sting hair, thorns etc., used against predatory animals. – Animals, on the other hand, know how to neutralize plant's self-defense properties. But then, they have to defend themselves against humans with a number of inherited tricks, often without a chance. – Humans, then, use plants and animals for their own personal goals, a fact which does not need to be demonstrated. And it is irrelevant that some farm plants [Nutzpflanzen] (such as crops and potatoes) and farm animals [Nutztiere] (cattle, goats, swine etc.) owe their wide distribution to humans. The last motive, anyway, was and is the self-interest and the struggle for life of the individual and collective I [Ich].

Such egoism is so big, that it cannot be contained within an individual's own class. It is well known, that plants take away foods and light from each other and that animals use others as food. In principle, we see the same in humans. This is particularly true of economics [Wirtschaftsleben], as has recently been pointed out by Naumann. Is it not the drive of the business man to outdo his competition or at least to be equally successful; his dealings with customers serve the same purpose. He would be a poor business man, besides, if he did otherwise! Similarly, national economy and world economy cannot and will not do without making good use of the struggle between different professions and different states. – Even intellectual intentions, at least as far as they are primarily professional, are not an exception. How does a young person (respectively parents or guardians) act, when determining which intellectually satisfying job to choose for life? – He inquires about his main interests and his best opportunities to have a good career, also in consideration and regard to the family. Only rarely does one ask seriously: "How can I serve humanity [Allgemeinheit] best with my properties and gifts?" Not even Kant could keep a utilitarian aspect totally away from his "Categorical Imperative", as Schopenhauer shows in detail in his "Über das Fundament der Moral".

Again, it must be pointed out in this context, that repeating these facts is not intended to be a demeaning critique. The egocentric attitude and the struggle for survival are extremely important for the creation and development of civilization, respectively culture. Under such an aspect, the consequences are a most blessed result for the community and the individual, even if not planned in the first place.

II.

Who, however, only values egoism, such as Stirner in his book "Der Einzige und sein Eigentum" and Nietzsche with his "Master-Human" model [Herrenmenschentum], "beyond good and bad", does not recognize that there is an altruism, also presenting a natural gift of normal human soul-life [Seelenleben]. Therefore, the empathy for right and fairness, compassion, sympathy, love – or what else we want to call it – first of all has to be recognized as a psychologically given fact and valued as such. If we don't do that or even suppress it, then we suppress and dominate human nature. And if there is someone arguing, that everything is based on genetics and education, then the following question has to be answered: "How come, altruism is inherited similarly to other human character traits [Seeleneigenschaft]?" Respectively: "Why do we target the education of the youth and the entire humankind in this direction and not in any other?", The most satisfying answer still is, that altruism is an empirically tested psychological fact of human soul, consequently we have to take this into account. "What, now, is altruism?" – It is the fact, that my own I [Ich] retracts totally behind something else, under certain conditions up to the point of self-destruction, and that egotistic motives do not come into force at all. An impressive example is animal protection out of sheer compassion, as understood by Schopenhauer and Richard Wagner and in the understanding of contemporary animal protection societies and animal protection legislation. – Those, who follow their altruistic inclinations, also have a personal satisfaction in doing so; this is another demonstration, that it might as well be an egotistic inclination. On the contrary: he, who with Kant wants only to accept reason or with Eduard von Hartmann cool-logical justice as the single correct motive for ethos, is as close to egoism and additionally sacrifices this phenomenon of human soul life.

Of course, similarly egoism is not without altruistic aspects, so is altruism not thinkable without any egoism. One example for many: Even though Christianity very correctly may be called the religion of love – a love disinterested in loving oneself as any religion of redemption, which can be defined best with the word: "Work out your own salvation" (Phil. 2:12). Important are also the words of Jesus: "So, whatever you wish that men would do to you, do to them" (Mt 7:12; Luke 6:31), also: "You shall love your neighbor as yourself" (Luke 10:27, following Lev 19:18). So, egoism is accepted as existing, and it is presupposed to be self-evident that everyone wants only good things from his neighbor and that everyone cares for himself. Do we want to regret this? – Surely, not easily. How would it be possible to provide for another being, i.e. to care for it in its struggle for survival, i.e. in his egotistic attitude, to protect it and to support it?! In particular, the interrelationship between altruism and egoism shows in the relationship of the individual as part of a community [Gesamtheit], may it be a professional organization, a political party, a village or an urban community, a national organization etc. Without doubt, there are people who submit their entire existence unto such a community, even sacrifice for it and in this way behave purely altruistic. As far as this community is concerned, it normally is resolute in struggling with other organizations or persons, i.e. it represents a collective egoism. Such a collective egoism, however, works well for the individual members of such a community in question and is in relation to it altruism as well. If such a positive effect of a specific organization is understood and used (and it has to be this way, otherwise such an organization under question would be useless), then the support of the community will play an important role for the individual as well. (F. Paulsen in his Ethics has expressed this and related issues in more detail).

As far as the evaluation of these two psychological, respectively ethical facts, as discussed above, is concerned, we have to mention the following: Only ethical skepticism seriously supports egocentric attitudes; but these are relatively few exemptions. Much larger is the number of those, who unconsciously make their own self the center of their interest. That this attitude is unavoidable and not necessarily to be criticized has been shown above. However, an exaggeration of egoism associated with endangering the ethos is obvious. These circumstances make it understandable that altruism carries a much higher recognition in public. Even those, who call love "sentimentality", routinely refrain from admitting their psychological shortcomings (and, indeed, these they are). Most people, however, possess, depending on their predisposition [Veranlagung], a serious will and confidence to be "just"", "good", "altruistic". The emotional, more or less unconscious higher esteem for altruism over egoism can be recognized by referring to witnesses in the history of ideas [Zeit- und Geistperioden], the first being the ideal, hoped to be realized finally in spite of the latter. Already the old Jewish prophet Isaiah refers to a future kingdom of peace, where the struggle for survival among animals and between animals and humans will have come to an end (Isa 11:6-9). Jesus similarly preaches about the coming of the kingdom of God, this means also the kingdom of love. It is easily understood when Paul in the first letter to the Corinthians, chapter 13, ascribes love a higher standing than faith and hope (verse 13) and attributes eternal existence to it (verse 8). In recent times, Kant, in postulating a moral demonstration of God's existence [Gottesbeweis], shows that he as well has the ideal of an exclusive rule of the good in the future. It should be mentioned that the favored idea in socialism about a "State of the Future", is an idea which without doubt bears a witness to ethical idealism and optimism.

What are now the most important consequences for social ethics?

1. Egoism and altruism are not necessarily incompatible ethical adversaries.

2. Egoistic mentality as a natural phenomenon is also a basic human right. If such a right is used reasonably (natural and healthy lifestyle, especially in regard nutrition, dressing, living and working conditions, also in a regulated and sufficient pay, not to forget also in the struggle for survival which can be regulated largely in justice and fairness), then it will be effective in wide circles and is – at least in its consequences – altruistic.

3. The psychological fact of egoistic attitude may also not be overlooked; and should not be without recognition. This requirement is easier to fulfill since its observation does not always result in personal harm. For example, what is spent in social welfare and in support and improvement of national strength [Volkskraft], returns with interest income, since the state and the

economy have a greatest interest to have trustworthy public servants, good workers, financially well off consumers, good development of the youth, and in general the wellbeing of the entire nation.

4. Now, egoism unfortunately quite often is overdone, a fact which is not the case with altruism. Therefore we have to care as much as possible for the belief in and the ideal of love, and to look optimistically at its future realization, e.g. with the faithful words of Goethe's "Faust": "Whoever strives hard enough, we will be allowed to redeem him", to redeem also from an exaggerated egoism. Caring for this ideal, of course, will never be without practical consequences. We may mention all activities in social care, in particular the support of the economically weak, not taking into account whether or not it will pay back (i.e. the care for the old and fragile; again also animal protection). The Christian churches, by the way, give enough references to work in the service of love.

Zwei ethische Grundprobleme in ihrem Gegensatz und in ihrer Vereinigung im sozialen Leben. *Ethik. Sexual- und Gesellschaftsethik* 1929, 5(5): 341-346

CHARACTER DICTATE OR FREEDOM OF THOUGHT? 1930

Thoughts about a liberal model of character education

Character [Gesinnung], in one way or the other, always is based on morally grounded judgment. Different from character is science, which does not accept value judgments as a basis of work. Of course, science can provide material for a character formation. And without doubt, this is very welcome. – But whenever it is done, it may also happen that no consequences are drawn or – whenever they are drawn – those may differ from person to person. (Germans and Frenchmen consider themselves to be traditional enemies. Some accept this without critique. Others probe deeper, but come to different conclusions: some want to solve the issue by means of war, others by means of agreement and understanding).

On the other hand, people try to influence science and culture and not always without success; they neglect scientifically proven facts of reality and start from a preconceived opinion. This sometimes happens even without a clear understanding of such a process. The mentioned transition from conviction to science (if such a transition is possible at all) only happens by eliminating objective reasoning in general or at least for a specific issue. Additionally, such a step becomes *a decorum* by covering it with an undeserved scientific cover.

Instead of presenting additional reflections, I want to review the practice of character education as it was, is today by far and large, and how it should be.

Let's look at first to the traditional disciplines of character education: religion, German literature, and history.

Traditional religion classes presuppose a firm understanding that religion, more than Christianity or even a denomination, has to form character, first in class, but then as well in later life. However, widely forgotten is that faith, in particular in Christian understanding, cannot be made obvious; also, the shortcomings of one's own conviction and the merits of other denominations are not admitted. The bible and other religious books preferably are used to select the passages which one likes, contradictions are not mentioned or manipulated according to the rule of Mephistopheles in Goethe's "Faust": "*Always be vigorous in hermeneutics. If you don't understand, you obscure*". Of course, we find similar misdeeds by those who are of different opinion; it is a misdeed, to breed arbitrary characters this way, which renders freedom of thought factually impossible (cf. article 135 of the German Constitution, which in no unclear terms guarantees all citizens of the Reich full freedom of faith and conscience).

German literature classes and history classes – especially since the times of the Romantic – are intended to instill the love of the fatherland and of the people, thereafter of the state and of the dynasty. Here are a few well known examples from a vast number of materials: "Right or wrong my country" says the Brit, while the German thinks that his country has to heal the world, and the Frenchman calls his country "La grande nation". Whether these character traits are desirable or not, shall not be judged here. Let's assume for a moment that those character traits are wanted. But then, what about the methods of character formation or character education? – One starts with an already existing character trait, but hides the subjective form of such a character under a so-called scientific cover and strictly rejects an unprejudiced logical review of such a questionable moral fiber. See, how Goethe lets his

"Faust" say: "*You are right; I don't find a trace of spirit, everything is broken in by training [Dressur]*". So, not freedom of thought, but trained, dictatorship of opinion (it has to be made very clear, that dictatorship may come from the political and pedagogical right, the middle, and the left). There are groups who accept these methods because of their effectiveness, irrespectively of their subjectivity and misconceived psychology. Thus it is very doubtful, if one can ever be content with the withdrawal of freedom of thought and its replacement by character dictate [Gesinnungsdiktatur].

But how should it be? The answer is self-evident from the preceding: Not brake-in by training, but liberalization, respectively "democratization", of character formation.

In classroom teaching it will work this way:

1. Do not teach predetermined subjective disposition [Gesinnung].
2. Strictly avoid the cover-up of a predetermined opinion with so-called objectivity and with so-called interactive teaching [Arbeitsunterricht].
3. Methodologically it is not acceptable to present only what is suitable and to suppress unsuitable facts, or to deny or to manipulate them at will.
4. Always consider different character attitudes [Gesinnungseinstellungen].
5. The benefits and shortcomings of different opinions and attitudes must be discussed. (Neither through a rosy glass, nor through a black one).
6. When you present your personal opinion, it must be in an impartial form. Also, one should forget to discuss problems associated with one's own position.
7. Instead of presenting biased character formation [Gesinnungsmacherei], students should be given the

opportunity to form their own opinion, respectively objective information should be given, so they may form their own character at a later date.

8. "Reason and science, people's greatest strength" never should be bypassed in the formation or review of an already existing character. Wrong is a rule, established by a newspaper in Munich: "Attitude first, thereafter reason". By the way, it would be satisfactory, if "reason" were to be allowed an objective review of character attitude.
9. One should not claim, that youth is only ready for authoritarian methods, not for methods of freedom, a position which might be contradicted by some. But, let it be! Sowing is always earlier than harvesting. The "Guidelines for Curricula at High Schools in Prussia" draw these consequences in methodological recommendations for various class teachings, expressively indicating that religious teaching in class has to be content with presenting material only, to be followed by student's *later* self-determination.
10. And if a new expected character is not developing, we should not forget, that had happened under the old method even more often. Additionally: a character acquired and formed by the self is better than one just accepted from others, also better than a childish or immature attitude towards character issues.

It is important to recognize that all disciplines in school teachings will support character formation. Mathematics, physics and chemistry teach exact precision and strict verification by avoiding any hint of moralizing. – Biology will improve much underdeveloped understanding of nature, get rid of old preconceptions, instill a love of nature, and respectively improve it. Music, painting, handcrafts and needlework favorably develop taste including aesthetics in character formation. – Gymnastics and sports satisfy human drives to wrestle in life. Additionally, they educate in camaraderie including the other team. Both establish reluctance to scuffle, hunger for war, and hatred among nations. In such a context, teaching foreign languages with cultural and historical aspects [Sachunterricht] is of eminent importance in character formation for the young, i.e. for the next generation of adults.

Gesinnungsdiktatur oder Gedankenfreiheit? Gedanken über eine liberale Gestaltung des Gesinnungsunterrichts. *Die neue Erziehung. Monatsschrift für entschiedene Schulreform und freiheitliche Schulpolitik*, 1930, 12: 200-202.
– An editorial footnote to this article reads: "We gladly publish this article because of its content, even though we ourselves are decidedly more in rejection to many issues – such as to the war. – Editors"

OUR DOUBTS ABOUT GOD. 1933

Subjective thoughts on the theme of another
(In Nr. 1, Jg. X, „Ethik“)

1. The truth cannot be known. Also, what we commonly call science does not give us true knowledge or actual recognition of truth. This I conclude from skepticism in old and new times, and from agnostic, positivist, and pragmatic schools of thought. When I ask myself: "What is truth?" (Pontius Pilate in John 18:38), I have to answer myself: "I know, that I don't know" (Socrates), "and I see that we *can* know nothing" (Goethe: Faust).

2. One thing, however, I do know with certainty is whether I am happy or not.

3. My happiness does not depend on money or possessions or other outward things, at least not in its deciding factors. Ultimately it always depends on something from within, something spiritual.

4. The greatest happiness of all things spiritual for me is always intertwined with love.

5. As love brings the greatest happiness, yes, even the greatest blessedness, my strivings cannot be selfish, but will unfailingly include essentially the wellbeing of others.

6. I judge my faith by what I know experientially, from a practical point of view. Two forms of belief are of interest to me: (a) Steadily changing opinions of the day, at that particular time called "common sense" [gesunder Menschenverstand]

and based on then available scientific views and perceptions (which are only just another form of belief).

– (b) The Christian religion.

7. (Ad 6a). What has called itself science at different times and in different places has surely quite often contributed to good fortunes for everyone, and thus to mine as well. In those cases, faith in dubious scientific knowledge is quite justified.

However, in the most difficult areas and most fateful moments of my aspirations for happiness, the presumed recognition of truth, the so-called scholarly truth, most often abandons me.

At times it even harms me, forcing me by civilization and technology into a realm of superficiality, away from the inner and spiritual life, on which my happiness and the happiness of the world depend. In this case, the true and good faith in presumed knowledge and truth becomes a false faith, a harmful superstition.

8. (Ad 6b). The Christian religion is as well a faith only. It possesses no less believability as the faith based on reasonable or scientific perceptions.

But above all: This faith makes me happy; for it gives me spiritual gifts, it is a religion of love. And as a religion of love it enables me to be a living and useful member of society at large.

9. The more "unadulterated" and "massive'", the more '"positive'" and decisive the Christian faith is; that is to say: the less dependent it is on ever changing opinions of the day, even as

they are paraded as exact scientific knowledge; the greater is the probability that it will bring happiness, – the more veracious it is.

10. "Our doubts about God?" – They have become null and void.

Unsere Zweifel an Gott. Subjektive Gedanken beim Thema eines Anderen (Nr. 1, Jg. X der ‚Ethik'). *Ethik. Sexual- und Gesellschaftsethik*. 1933, 10(1): 115-116.
– Jahr refers to an article „Unsere Zweifel an Gott" by Luise Hartmann-Rücklos in *Ethik. Sexual- und Gesellschaftsethik. Organ des Ethikbundes*, 1933, 10(1): 28-33.

CHILD AND TECHNOLOGY. 1933

"Ethik" Nr. 9 published the article "The Gratitude of Children" [Kindesdankbarkeit] by O. Craemer. This essay describes two characteristics of today's youth. One is “being without history” [Geschichtslosigkeit], the other “technical attitudes and aptitudes”. I will address the latter, using photography as a typical example.

Is the child of today indeed technically more mature? Many elementary school students, yes, even pre-school children, own cameras and most eagerly shoot pictures. Nothing more is required of them, than to "shoot away" and to advance the film. These are technical achievements, but minor ones. – And what about comprehension? The fewest children are aware of the technical properties, advantages and disadvantages of a camera. They know even less about the physical and chemical principles involved in the development of a picture. They don't know why lenses are used. They know nothing about refractions of different light rays, the magnifications with proper combination of lenses, nor the simultaneous use of different kinds of glass. The terms "light-meter", "focal length" and "focus" are meaningless to them. Just as the optical and mechanical basis of a camera in general, and the shutter in particular, remain unknown. Neither are they knowledgeable about negative or positive chemical treatments, or how to judge their completion. They are ignorant of the properties of “argentic bromide”, resp. “silver chloride” in regards to multicolored lights, as well as the reductive strength of developers or the workings of the fixatives. There is much more that they know little about. The fact, that the child does not even regard any of this as wonderful is significant. The child only "wonders, when something does not work immediately"

(O. Craemer). – One might object that they do not need to know, that it presents unnecessary ballast. It is sufficient that the photo shop should know. – Admitted. But one cannot speak of an exceptional technical attitude and aptitude of today's youth compared to the past, in view of their great void in technical and scientific background.

What is left? Youth takes advantage of the readily available appliances without the necessary technical background knowledge. The truly technical advances of today rest with grownups, – with the specialist, who produced the tool, enabling an untrained hand to achieve such goals without difficulty. One is reminded of Faust's citation: "I do not find a trace of a Spirit, everything is only dressage."

Several animals are on a corresponding level with these technical skills. (I emphasize, that a comparison with animals does not lower humanity.) In olden times, at the fair, I could see poor little monkeys, which could, besides other tricks, aim a gun and pull a trigger – very similar to a child, who aims and shoots with a camera. Other examples are clever elephants, who can drop a coin, handed to them, and retrieve treats.

In view of this knowledge one realizes, that the danger of great superficiality associated with technical gadgetry and coupled with an exaggerated self-confidence, threatens our youth, and in my opinion avoidance of this danger is rarely attempted. "Too early do they regard themselves as accomplished and all-knowing, and dismiss parents and their outdated views – (for) especially, when void of understanding, easy words find easy flow" (O. Craemer). And yet, they owe all the technical progress to their parents – yes, everything.

Do these events indicate a turning tide? If so, it is not a turn for the best. In reality, it is hardly such. Often, the cause can be found with the fathers, who are stuck in book-taught professions or offices. They forgot that they themselves did play with technical things: the rifle and cannon, the building block, model trains and steamers, with mechanical toys and whatever else they had, and they understood those techniques just like the youth of today, perhaps a bit more. As a consequence of this their professions further have not kept a pace with technical development and the toys of the times. This explains the all too prevalent overestimation of children's technical abilities. In my personal observations this is a bit different among craftsmen and laborers: These individuals have greater technical understanding (and ability in practical usage), which ranks higher than their children's and therefore more are valued than childish play.

I hardly need to reiterate: Today's youth, in my opinion, are not more advanced in technology, but are as any youth would have been in similar circumstances and times. If in a very few cases they could be, it is only because the adults of today gave their children greater room to play with technology and at the same time introduced them to the technical aspects of their surroundings.

This holds true, not only for children with photography, but all the other technical toys as well, such as the bicycle and its substitutes: the scooter, radio, model airplane, accessories for the car business and whatever else happens to be fashionable.

And the "moral consequence" of these observations? Briefly: a change in the relationship between child and adult on the basis of supposedly self-earned technical skills by the child seems far afield, and so are the educational measures (resp. the removal of such), if based on this erroneous opinion.

Kind und Technik. *Ethik. Sexual- und Gesellschaftsethik.* 1933, 9(6): 400-402.
– A response to an article by O. Craemer, Kindesdankbarkeit, *Ethik. Sexual- und Gesellschaftsethik. Organ des Ethikbundes,* 1933, 9(5): 304-313

LIFE AFTER DEATH. 1934

(Arranged from "Didactia magna" by J. A. Comenius)

> In this year, the year of Hindenburg's passing and the twentieth anniversary of the beginning of the war with its great outpouring of death, this Year's Memorial-day stirs in us especially serious thoughts. But thoughts of dying visit us all, independently of current events. In this context it is interesting to leaf through "The Little Book about Life after Death" by scientist and philosopher G. Th. Fechner (who precisely 100 years ago became Professor of Physics in Leipzig). (The little book is easily read and captivating and not too long), and many, who read it do not know that these thoughts of Fechner had found nearly identical expression by J. A. Comenius two hundred years ago. Comenius, Bishop of the Bohemian Brethren, a branch of the Herrenhuter Bruedergemeinde, was one of the great pedagogues of the new times. From his pedagogic masterpiece "Didactica magna" the following thoughts about life after death have been assembled.

"Everyone's life and its dwelling place are threefold: the womb, the earth, the heavens: in the first we are only given life, endowed with movement and the beginnings of consciousness, in the second life, movement, consciousness with the beginnings of knowledge, in the third limitless completion of all.

The first life is a preparation for the second, the second for the third, the third goes off in itself without end. … The first and second dwelling may be comparable to workshops, where the body gets ready for usefulness in the following life; the third dwelling place will bring the completion and enjoyment of both." – "Our first life rests in the lap of our mothers. But what for? For its own advantage? Far from it. It is only concerned, that the little body be made a suitable dwelling place and instrument of the soul, for the comfortable use in the life-after to be enjoyed under the sun. As soon as this is accomplished, we break into the light, because nothing further can happen in this darkness. Similarly, life under the sun is nothing but a preparation for the eternal life, in so far that the soul in the service of the body has earned what is needed for the future life." – "Just as we can be sure that the stay in the mother's womb is preparation for life in the body, it is just as sure, that the stay of the body is a preparation for the life, which will follow this and will last forever. Happy is he, who leaves the mother's womb well formed! A thousand times happier he, who carries a well adorned soul from here along with him."

"This world is nothing more than a garden, our storehouse, our school. There is a beyond, to which we graduate after dismissal from this school, the eternal academy." – "The descriptions attributed to this life let us understand, that it is only a preparation for the other life. This life is called way, walk, gate, expectancy, we are called strangers, pilgrims, tenants, in hopes of a different state, one that will be permanent. (Cf.1 Gen. 47, 9. Psalm 39, 13, Job 7,12. Luke 12, 36.)"

However: "The passage from the first life to the second, and from the second to the third, is tight and painful, but in both cases only the clothing and wraps are left behind (which are only secondary there, but here the prison of the body), just as from a broken eggshell the young one appears."

Vom Leben nach dem Tode *Ethik. Sexual- und Gesellschaftsethik.* 1934, 11(2): 50-51

THREE STUDIES ON THE FIFTH COMMANDMENT. 1934

I.

The 5th Commandment as an Expression of the Moral Law

How can we do good? – The so called "Golden Rule" gives answer to this question: Whatever you want the people do unto you, the same do unto them (Matthew 7:12; Luke 6:31). Kant's "Categorical Imperative": Act only according to the maxim whereby you can, at the same time, will that it should become a universal law, – this basically means the same. – But are these and similar formulations present not only just a formal criterion for "good" action. The motive, disregarding such a criterion, could just be blatant egoism, a so called contract on reciprocity: Do nothing to me, so that, in return, I will do nothing to you (Schopenhauer hints at this in his "Grundlage der Moral").

If we are aware that love is the fulfillment of the moral law (Romans 18:10), we indeed are already one step ahead: We know the motive. But we do not yet know the concrete content of the moral law; we don't know what specifically to do or not to do. Here, Schopenhauer, gives as helping hand: He says that the best, the most concrete specification of the moral act is the sentence: Neminem laede, imo omnes, quantum potes juva! (Don't hurt anyone, but help everyone, as far as you possibly can!)

More than two millennia before Schopenhauer, the 5th commandment already provides this insight, and, in fact, in a broader perspective than benefit or harm, namely under the perspective of sanctity of life and life's manifestations. Therefore the command: "You shall not kill!" We know from Jesus that the 5th commandment does not only prohibit killing, but prohibits all wrong deeds against others, even the bad word, even the bad thought. This means: He not only forbids the malicious or careless destruction of life, but also everything that, in one way or another, may hinder or trouble life. Luther in his Catechism has made it clear, that the 5th Commandment has to be understood not only in a negative, but as well in a positive way. – Consequently, the 5th commandment is a very good expression of what it means to be morally and practically good.

II.
The Duty of Self-Preservation

When talking about moral duties, normally we mean duties towards other people in the first place. Routinely we do not consider that each person has moral duties towards oneself as well, and that those duties are of immense importance. Christian religion expressively mentions those moral duties of everyone towards oneself. That basically applies to the 5th commandment as well: "You shall not kill". In this sense – "You shall not harm or hurt anyone's body or life, rather help and support him/her in all distresses of body and life, wherever you can"[1] – in the first place, meaning the life of our "neighbor". The final consequence, however, is: in a Christian perspective every human life as such is morally "sacred" – including one's own life. Preservation of life – and one's own life not excluded – is a duty. And destruction and harm – again, including one's own life – is a moral sin. "Don't you know, that you are God's temple and that God's spirit dwells

[1] Cf. Luther's explanation of the 5th Commandment, German and Latin

in you? You shall keep God's temple sacred and not destroy it." (following 1. Corinthian 3:16-17).

How should these moral duties, expressed in the 5th commandment towards one's own life, be applied in real life's practice? By not taking one's own life, not shortening it, not harming or endangering it, not weakening one's health by unchastity, excesses in eating and drinking, heavy anger, frivolous foolhardiness and daredevilry, etc.. Particularly important is the protection of sexual virtue and the avoidance of abuse of alcoholic drinks. – As far as the first one is concerned, the judgment of the New Testament is particularly clear: "If you have loose sex, you sinfully harm your own life" (following 1. Corinthian 6:18). But not only is it a duty to oneself to abstain from fornication, but also avoid anything, which might lead to unchastity: indecent looks, unclean or double talk, dancing, dresses etc. – As far as alcoholism is concerned, the Christian attitude is based on recognizing that "wine kills many people" (Sirach 31:30), i.e. alcohol endangers life and brings great dangers to health.

Are the duties towards one's own life in conflict with duties towards the neighbor? – That is not necessarily the case. On the contrary: Whoever fulfills the duties towards oneself, avoids many forms of harm to other people. That can be shown in regard to the already mentioned issues of sex and alcohol: Who falls into dependency and unchastity, endangers and weakens oneself physically and spiritually. Venereal diseases threaten as well. Weakness and disease cause the victim to be more and more a burden to the community, harming everyone. If one has offspring, they also are harmed, as they may inherit a weak or sick nature, causing additional burdens and harm to the community. Whoever protects his own life in this regard, he fulfills one's duty also towards the community.

Similar with alcohol: Those, who are dependent on consuming alcohol, may eventually expose themselves to severest physical and spiritual dangers. And thus does not only harm oneself, but one's family as well, one's offspring, one's country, and one's race[2]. And again: If one protects oneself in this regard against harm, one does, at the same time, good to one's neighbor, actually to one's entire country.

III.
The Bioethical Imperative

The 5th Commandment admonishes "Thou shalt not kill". Now, the term killing always means killing something which is alive. Living entities, however, are not only humans, but animals and plants as well. Because the 5th commandment does not expressively prohibit the killings of humans exclusively, should it not logically be applied towards animals and plants as well?

But are animals and plants so close to us, that we must recognize and treat them actually as our neighbors? – When we review publications in modern science, we find immediately similar studies of humans and animals as subjects in research, not only in physiology, but also in psychology. Such equal treatment today is not reserved, as already mentioned, for humans; similar methods are applied in the field of animals, and – as there is a comparative anatomical-zootomic research – similarly very interesting comparisons are made be-

[2] Alcohol is "a mean enemy of our race", cf. the brochure with this title by Wilhelm John, reviewed in no. 2 of *Ethik*.

tween the human soul and animal soul[3]. Yes, even the beginnings of plant psychology are recognizable – the most well-known among them are G. Th. Fechner[4] in the past, R. H. Francé[5], and Ad. Wagner[6] at present – thus modern psychology includes all living beings in its research. Given this, it is only consequent, that E. Eisler[7], in summarizing, speaks of a Bio-Psychik.

From Bio-Psychics, it is only a small step to Bio-Ethics, i.e. to the assumption of moral duties not only towards humans, but towards all living beings. In fact, bioethics is not a discovery of today. Montaigne[8] – the only early representative of modern ethics of sentiment – already grants all living beings an entitlement of being treated based on moral principles: We owe justice to humans; mildness and mercy towards all living beings, capable of having a benefit from that. Similarly, Herder[9] requires that humans – following the model of God in their sentiments – put themselves into the place of every living being and feel with it, as much as it requires. Those lines of reasoning are continued by the theologian Schleiermacher[10], who calls it immoral, to destroy life and formation – wherever they are, i.e. including animals and plants – without a reasonable argument for doing so. Therefore philosopher

---

[3] Among recent publication in animal psychology especially recommendable are: Sommer, Tierpsychologie, Leipzig 1925. – Alverdes, Tierpsychologie, Leipzig 1925.

[4] G. Th. Fechner, Nana oder das Seelenleben der Pflanze [1848; 5th ed. 1921]

[5] R. H. Francé, Pflanzenpsychologie als Arbeitshypothese der Pflanzenphysiologie, Stuttgart 1909.

[6] Ad. Wagner, Die Vernunft der Pflanze, Dresden 1926.

[7] R. Eisler, Das Wirken der Seele, Stuttgart 1908.

[8] Montaigne, Essays.

[9] Herder, Ideen zur Geschichte der Philosophie der Menschheit.

[10] Schleiermacher, Philosophische Sittenlehre (Kirchmann 1870).

Krause[11], a contemporary of Schleiermacher, requests that every living being has to be valued as such and not be destroyed without reason. Because they all, plants and animals like humans, have an equal right; but not totally equal, each only as a precondition to reach its destiny. Schopenhauer[12] in particular refers to the Indian realm of reasoning, stressing compassion as the most important motive of his ethics, and requesting it also for animals. It was Richard Wagner, strongly influenced by Schopenhauer and a passionate animal friend, who made those thoughts commonly known.

As far as animals are concerned, the moral request has become obvious for a long time[13], at least in that form, not to harm animals without purpose. With plants it is different. However in regard to new biological and biopsychic knowledge (see above), also regarding the various thoughts mentioned above from Montaigne, Herder, Schleiermacher and Krause, moral duties towards plants become visible. For purely sentimental-poetic argumentation such recognition is nothing new. Think of Goethe, who has Faust call plants his brothers, or of Richard Wagner's Parsifal: In pious devotion people, at least on Good Friday, protect weeds and flowers in the meadow by walking carefully, in order not to hurt them. More seriously we have to consider the plant-ethical reflections of a quite matter-of-fact Eduard von Hartmann[14]. In an article on flower luxury he writes about a picked blossom: "She is a deadly wounded organism, the colors of which are not harmed yet, a still living and smiling head, separated from

[11] K. Chr. Fr. Krause, Das System der Rechtsphilosophie (Röder, Leipzig 1874).

[12] Schopenhauer, Über das Fundament der Moral.

[13] The most comprehensive book in this area still is Bregenzer, Tierethik, Bamberg 1894.

[14] Psychological preconditions are discussed in W. von Schnehen, Ed. von Hartmann und die Pflanzenpsycholgie, Stuttgart 1908.

its stem. – When, however, I put the rose into a glass of water, I cannot help myself but fighting the thought, that man has murdered a flower life, in order to enjoy the dying process by an eye, heartless enough to not sense the unnatural death under the appearance of life"[15]. The requirements of plant ethics, leading to such recognition, are quite clear.

As far as the potential realization of such moral duties to all living beings is concerned, it might seem utopian. But we may not ignore, that moral obligations towards a living being related to its "need" (Herder), respectively to its "destiny" (Krause). It appears, that needs of animals seem much less in number, and their content less complex than those of people. This applies even more to plants, so that moral obligations to them should produce less complication than those to animals, as they are lower (if not conceptually, so nevertheless practically). Here also comes the principle of struggle for survival into play, a principle which also modifies our moral obligations towards fellow humans at no low scale. Within these limits there always will be enough possibilities for bioethical actions. Paragraphs for animal protection in penal codes of various cultivated nations[16] give guidance in this regard. Confer in particular the new German Reich Animal Law. As far as plant ethics is concerned, we are guided by our sentiment, which will hinder us to pick flowers and then throw them away carelessly shortly thereafter, or to deadhead plants with a walking stick, or when we find it disgusting to recognize the blind destructive impulse of rowdy lads in breaking the heads of small trees along the road. Also, excessive flower luxury –

---

[15] Ed. Von Hartmann, Der Blumenluxus, 1885.

[16] For the first time, material has been extensively collected and reviewed in R. von Hippel, Die Tierquälerei in der Strafgesetzgebung des In- und Auslandes, Berlin 1891.

in learning from Ed. von Hartmann – is not morally refined and can be avoided.

In sum, the universal realm of authority of the 5th Commandment is clear and demands application to all forms of life. A transcription of the 5th Commandment results in the Bioethical Imperative: "Respect every living being in principle as an end in itself and treat it, if possible, as such!"

Drei Studien zum 5. Gebot. *Ethik. Sexual- und Gesellschaftsethik.* 1934, 11(4): 183-187

FAITH IN THE HEREAFTER AND ETHICS IN CHRISTIANITY, 1934

A Post-Easter Contemplation

When we consciously listen to the word "Christ"-ianity, we realize that the belief in Christ is an essential of Christianity. On closer examination we find that this faith concerns particularly the risen Christ. We don't have to prove that here. Only one single, but very instructive example is necessary: In Athens, when Paul preached among a gathering of philosophers, his core message was "Jesus and the resurrection" (Acts 17:18, 31). And in a letter to the Corinthians he expresses the following: A Christianity without the risen Christ is no Christianity. (cf.1. Cor 15:14 and 17) The belief in the Easterly resurrection is at the same time a belief in the resurrection of those, who were saved in Christ. That means: Faith in Christ is a faith in the life-to-come.[1]

On the other hand, Christianity is highly valued as a religion of love, and rightfully so. Again, there is no need for proof here: In the New Testament, time and again, the commandment of brotherly love and love-of-your-neighbor, yes, even love-of-your-enemy confronts us, and from the very beginning until this day love is extended and practiced in the most dire situations. Especially praiseworthy in the history of charity is the work in the education of youth, the help given to the aging, the care for the poor, for the sick and frail, for the fallen and abandoned. This work also raised others into such

[1] Cf. „Vom Leben nach dem Tode", 11(2), p. 50

useful service – their teacher long since forgotten and possibly even disdained.

During the last centuries, the Christian belief in the here-after has experienced more doubt and rejection than ever before. In contrast to this, the Christian ethic has held its ground and is widely respected, even when a belief in the Easter-message is wanting. One can understand this drift away from a belief in the here-after [Jenseits] and towards Christian ethics as a sign of the times. However, it would be inappropriate to separate the one from the other, because they do depend on each other.

On the one hand, the belief in the here-after is well-founded in ethics: when we know the commandment of God, which regards life as sacred[2], it is an obvious conclusion to believe that God would, in accordance with his commandment, regard and treat his creatures as holy and not let them expire in death. This is one of the ethic roots of the belief in the here-after. Another one follows: in the end, all good will finally find its just rewards, likewise all evil will reap its rewards. Plainly, this is not the rule in this life and it becomes an axiom of faith in goodness and its final victory in the life-to-come.

Just as the belief in the here-after leans heavily on ethical considerations, so do ethics bear the stamp of a belief in the here-after: Ethics derives great strength and confidence from the expectation of the victory of good, which the belief-in-the-beyond confirms.

From this we learn: Whoever cannot rightly accommodate the Christian belief in the here-after – and that includes more Christians than the churches are willing to confess – but is cognizant of the value of Christian ethics, he may via ethics

[2] Cf. „Drei Studien zum 5. Gebot", 11(4), p. 183

come to a deeper understanding and higher appreciation of the belief in the beyond.

Jenseitsglaube und Ethik im Christentum. *Ethik. Sexual- und Gesellschaftsethik* 1934, 11(5): 217-218.
– In footnotes 1 and 2 Jahr refers to his articles „Life after Death" and "Three Studies on the 5th Commandment", in this edition pages 73 to 75 and 77 to 84.

THE ETHICAL-SOCIAL IMPORTANCE OF SUNDAY. 1934

The weekly rest and holiday in Caucasian-occidental western culture comes from the Bible. Yet, the true meaning of that day remains unclear to the followers. When asked, what do they answer? "Sunday is to remember the resurrection of Jesus". This is true, indeed. But Christians should never forget this and remember such an important fact of faith all week long. Another answer might be: "A work-free day on the weekend is a reminder of the completion of God's creation". This is true as well. But the believer should not forget his Creator during the week. Or: "On Sundays you are supposed to hear God's word and somehow serve him". This is also correct, but one should not necessarily need a work-free day for that; it can also be done on weekdays. In some instances work is regarded as a service to God and the Sunday rest might even prove to be a hindrance in our service to God. What is important?: To not work and to not to ask others to work.

From an idealistic point of view, to be freed from work seems strange. Work is indispensable in three ways: it is a necessary instrument of love, or in more modern language, of a conscientious social duty. It is furthermore a practical necessity. And lastly: to work with sense and purpose is a joy, – to produce value [Werte schaffen] creates a sense of value [Wertgefühl].

Sadly, this threefold benefit of work is often lost, because love – the sense of social duty – is missing. Instead we find selfishness in greed and thirst for pleasure. Even though the government in Germany today tried a change, it remains true that humanity as a whole stays the same. Such selfishness only knows its own interests. Concerns for others are unimportant and conveniently ignored, unless these concerns serve one's own advantage as well. Such a feeling creates mistrust and combativeness, so the blessings of work are lost. In this way people turn work into some sort of fight, and that sadly means brother fights against brother.

Such a struggle does not lose its rancor just when it parades as "friendly competition". In this way people create in their work thorns and thistles, far worse than any field could grow. The beads of sweat created by this man-made fight burn and corrode far more than those, work alone might produce. Those man-made burdens are much heavier than those of other daily and natural events – to the believers these are god-sent fates (Gen 3:18, 19), which serve man for the best in the end (Rom 8:18, 28). Under these circumstances the joys of work may embitter people or even be completely taken away.

Here the weekly work-free day is of great help. When work is at rest, so are greed and envy; even though they still exist. When work is at rest, the fight for existence, for survival and the daily bread rests as well, – this fight which pits man against man instead of overcoming common burdens in a united way. On those days a Sunday-mood gives peace to all spirits. On such a day of peace one can hear more clearly the words of love, which otherwise are drowned out by the restless rush of the world. One's own heart can easily find the way to the other, also the people and spirits come closer to each other. Even if love at first has only the power to stop certain actions – then there is a multitude of actions that should cease out of compassion and love – it is a very great cultural benefit, – for the ethical culture, for the "social" culture[1].

It is a special benefit if such a day of rest is not restricted to a small group of people. It is not only for the rich but also the poor, not only far the master but also for the servant and maid, not only for the entrepreneur but also for the workforce. Even the poor work-animal needs a day of rest. It is a blessing for all of humankind not just for those following the Bible; regardless of the Christian Bible it is a blessing to every living thing. Founding a day of rest for everyone, regardless of their rank, social or economic standing, or faith, from a historic point of view is an extraordinary achievement of greatest ethical and social value.

The fact that the believer recognizes that such a social institution, i.e. the day of rest is based on God's revelation, on God's love, and that respecting the day of rest as one of the first (in third or fourth place) commandments, shines a bright light on his faith. This light is even brighter for not being an afterthought or an adaptation from another faith, but an essential original thought from within. And even though it was formally ordered by government (Emperor Konstantin in the year 321 after Christ decreed the first Sunday law), the thought itself originated in the Bible and believers had long since observed it in their small circles. If the concept had not first arisen there and been established, humankind might up to this very day be without any holiday, any armistice in the harsh fight for existence – by people themselves robbed of any holiness –, day in day out, week for week, year in year out, '"until he returns to earth, from which he was taken"'

[1] Also: "It is not only for ethical reasons, to respect the Sunday holiday, much more ... also for health'"; cf. Abderhalden "Die Bedeutung der Sonntagsruhe auf dem Lande" [The Meaning of Sunday Rest], in "Ethik", 10(4), p. 241

(Gen 3,19). Thus the social-ethical importance of the weekly holiday is significant and confirms at the same time the biblical source of the day of rest until this very day.

Die sittlich-soziale Bedeutung des Sonntags. *Ethik. Sexual- und Gesellschaftsethik* 1934, 10(6): 361-363

DOUBTS ABOUT JESUS? 1934[1]

In the person of Parsifal the "pure fool" [reiner Tor] model is incarnated. Similar thoughts arise from two of the Beatitudes in the New Testament: "Blessed are the pure in heart!" (Matth. 5:8); "Blessed are the poor in spirit!" (Matth. 5:3). Further, we remember the story of Christ reminding his disciples to follow the example of children, innocent and free of intricacy (Mark 10:15). In harmony with this, Wagner opposes vehemently the intellectuality, which he sees as taking on an erroneous path. He notes especially the new directions of the natural sciences, which declare the world consists of "matter and energy" exclusively, which contemptuously regard philosophy and religion as rudiments of the past, also deny any form of religious intuition. It would, however, be quite erroneous to regard Wagner's premise as: "Despise any reason and science!" His ire is not directed at the sciences, but at rationalistic one-sidedness and at materialistic distortions. Pure knowledge is of incomparably high value to him. And how can we achieve this? Through love which in Schopenhauer's pessimistic worldview – shared by Wagner – can only manifest itself in compassion. "Knowledgeable by compassion" [durch Mitleid wissend].

What about Parsifal's development in this regard? Parsifal's first step on this road is to be able to feel pain for having killed a swan in haughtiness. (Wagner, a follower of Schopenhauer, considered animals and people identical in nature [wesensverwandt].) When led inside the Temple of the Grail, Parsifal is deeply moved to see the unhappy Grail-king Amfortas lying on his bed of pain. As he learns in Klingsor's

[1] A contemplation following Richard Wagner's 'Parsifal'; cf. 'Our Doubts about God', 10(2), Nov./Dec. 1935, p. 115.

enchanted garden, he gains wisdom in understanding Amfortas' pain, i.e. the greatest pain in spiritual anguish suffering from guilt; he gains this highest wisdom by empathy and compassion. Now: "through compassion did he become knowing" and wise [durch Mitleid wissend].

The meaning of the above is clear – also for religion: It is not intellectualism in a one-sided derailed form, but "the power that compassion imparts to love'" [des Mitleids Liebesmacht], which leads us to the knowledge of truth: "Knowing through compassion". It also applies to the truth of religion: "To love God is the sweetest wisdom" (Jesus Sirach 1,14).

Can we likewise philosophically conceptualize that, which Wagner found through intuition in the arts? Love, clothed in compassion and directed to the wellbeing of others, yes, of all, is a curious fact of human "emotion" [Gefühlsleben]. To feel and to exercise an all-embracing love represents highest happiness and blessedness, as far as we know. The reality of such happiness stands up to all doubts; for, whoever feels happy, he is also happy. Here appearance and reality are identical. Does it even make sense to try to differentiate between them? Here, love is very well suited to be the foundation for further knowledge, the knowledge of truth in religious intuition.

The foregone seems to portray the religious worldview of "Parsifal" as a Buddhist religion based on compassion, by way of Schopenhauer's intuits. Schopenhauer regards this kind of religiosity as to be contrary to Christianity. That, however, is incorrect. Yes, the highly valued compassion takes us to the very center of Christian thought. Christianity holds love (compassion being part of it) in the highest esteem, above what may itself call cognition, knowledge or wisdom (1 Cor.

13). Nietzsche, having a different understanding of Christianity, severely attacks Wagner and 'Parsifal' and herewith verifies that we are truly dealing with Christian principles. It remains true for the Christian religion: Love (shown as empathy, as compassion) is foundation and premise for any realization of the truth.

Exclusively and singularly it is love that determines our relationship to Jesus. His suffering is a "love-offering" [Liebesopfer] out of mercy and compassion. After his death on the cross he mystically approaches his followers through "compassion's power of love" [des Mitleids Liebesmacht] at the Holy Supper, which now has become a "meal of love". This is in keeping with the love between man saved and the savior, so that heavenly voices can sound in the Temple-of-the-Grail:

"Take my body,
take my blood ,
for the sake of our *love!"*

Here, too, love means knowledge. And, whoever through love has found certainty that Jesus is the bearer of salvation [Bringer des Heils], he has conquered all doubt,

"blessed in love, blessed in faith".

Zweifel an Jesus. Eine Betrachtung nach Richard Wagner's „Parsifal". *Ethik. Sexual- und Gesellschaftsethik* 1934, 10 (6): 363-364 – In footnote 1 Jahr refers to his article "Our Doubts about God", in this edition pages 65 to 67.

ETHICAL REFLECTIONS ON INTER-CHRISTIAN QUARRELS, 1935

Christianity split into hundreds of directions, be it denominations, independent churches, sects, congregations and the likes. That surely is regrettable. Also, this splintering is not in to the spirit of Christ. However, such multifaceted expression makes sense from a psychological point of view. Genuine religiosity is a highly personal matter of the individual human soul. The more adherent and intensive the religious devotion, the more likely the deciding gradations of differences amongst the various people and groups will turn out, so that no two people's inner believes are alike. Perhaps the many forms of belief attest to the strength of the religion and, from that point of view, could be a good sign.

It is mandatory that the richness of forms of belief must not cause religious unrest among the Christians. Such danger is very real and, from the past up to the present, the same thing always happens: The Christian churches, which are uniquely pioneering in their works of charity, a model for all of modern culture, show a terribly short supply of this love in the behaviors toward each other in matters of differing religious opinions. Instead of the peace, that Christ expects, we find intolerance, disharmony, quarrel and dispute – one could even call this the norm. It need not be and should not be so.

Take note. As the multifaceted Christian views can be a positive sign, an objective disagreement or a fight – if you wish to call it that – could be useful and necessary. Only, this "fight" among Christians must adhere to Christian standards and a Christian spirit. That takes a lot. I will discuss three important points of Christian bearings on this fight, which should be observed:

1. *It is preferable to keep an eye on what unites us prior to that which divides us*[1].

Central to any Christian church form is this important question: How do we differ from other Christians? In the evangelical state-church [Staatskirche] this question is: What makes us different from other protestant free-churches and sects? How does our view differ from the Catholics? These questions should be very similar in the free-churches and Catholics. Quite a few catechisms devote a special section to this. These subjects are part of school and university examinations. To know these differences is important – one should know what makes one's church special – but it is much more important to know what we hold in common. And the common ground consists of much more than a casual gleaning would show.

2. *When dealing with differences one should not exaggerate the other's conceptual weaknesses and remain silent about the positives.*

Everything done by man is incomplete and it is not at all difficult to find the shortcomings of it, especially if one tries. This applies to all religious conceptions and their expressions – including the Christian. In other words, it is always somehow possible to find weaknesses and a lack of completeness in the theories and practices of other Christians – with a tendency to exaggerate these. When at the same time you conveniently say nothing about their good

[1] Cf. the efforts of the 'German Christians' movement in Thuringia [Thüringer "Kirchenbewegung Deutsche Christen] and a supporting review by Erich Friedel in *Ethik* 11(5), p. 213 ff.: "Church of Love" [Die Kirche der Liebe].

points, it proves tactically effective: you can deal them a blow. Such tactics are no doubt very human. But this is totally incompatible with Christian ethics.

3. *True mistakes or actual weaknesses in the other's belief should be rejected, however, in a most objective manner and without impassioned agitation.*

   To speak metaphorically, one may not overlook a white or even change it into a black. Under no circumstances would truth and justice permit it. Clearly for the same reason a black may not be overlooked or covered with white. I must repeat: mistakes must be verified beyond any doubt. One has to be very cautious with negative critique; especially in the area of religion – also the Christian religion – the danger is great that one may judge from a presumed truth and justice, i.e. one misjudges. Indeed, if a true denial is justified and necessary, then it should always proceed in a most objective manner and without any impassioned agitation, that is to say: without any hint of coarseness, without animosity and odiousness, without arrogance and know-it-all, without strife and being over-critical, and without any desire to score mistakes.

Finally, one must become aware that one's own religion has shortcomings and weaknesses, for which a lenient judgment is taken for granted. Such a consciousness should suffice to take on a kinder judgment towards the shortcomings of others.

Ethische Betrachtungen zu innerchristlichen Glaubenskämpfen. *Ethik. Sexual- und Gesellschaftsethik. Organ des Ethikbundes* 1935, 12(2): 58-61

FAITH AND WORKS: OPPOSITION AND ALLIANCE. 1935

The philosopher Kant states that good will alone is good enough. This means: one can rightfully affix the designation of good only to the will. In everyday speech that would mean: All depends on the will, the heart, the character [Gesinnung]. Works of people are good, if attitudes, from which they come, are good.

However, one cannot look into another person's heart. Even in reviewing one's own work, one often errs about one's true motive: one usually believes in one's good intentions, but this quite often is far from being true. In practical life, most of the time we will not reflect from character onto deeds, rather from deeds onto character. (Matth. 7:16, 20: "By their fruits you shall know them!") The same is in Kant's "Categorical Imperative": "Act in such a manner, that the maxims of your action can as well serve as a principle for a common law!" This is a call to good actions, whereby the good result of the deeds is not determined by character [Gesinnung], but by very real things, i.e. common goods. On the one hand: the intentions are what count, on the other: it is the actions. This appears contradictory, but is not. Of course, an honest good will is the condition for actions, if they indeed can be called good. But on the other hand, even if the deed logically comes after the intention, the deed is the yardstick for measuring intention. There are no truly good intentions if good actions do not follow, just as no truly good action can be without good intent. Intentions and deeds, or deeds and intentions are on equal footing and are inseparable in practice, even if not so in logic.

In applying these facts to Christianity, one would use faith for compassion – in place of actions one would use deeds – thus: faith and deeds, deeds and faith, both are practically inseparable. This fact has never been unknown to churches. At times, however the one or the other, faith or deeds, was regarded as more important, and this led to all kinds of misunderstandings among those, who differed in opinions about the greater importance of either. The more one side exaggerated; the surer the opposite side would exaggerate as well, this happening consciously or subconsciously. From a human point of view such fractions are quite understandable. But it is regrettable because both disunited parties could quite well have found common ground.

Take for example *Catholic thinking in the Middle Ages*. Never were they taught that character [Gesinnung] does not count and therefore, e.g., it is not necessary to believe in God. However, doing was more emphasized than faith, which is understandable: others can be deceived by a presumed or supposed kind character disposition – and even the self. That should be avoided, in those days and today as well. Even if good and right intentions are truly present, but too weak, easily disabled by fear or laziness or any other such hindrance, that likewise is not right. A focus on the importance of deeds does not disrespect the importance of character disposition. A misunderstanding did arise here: one could do this or that, e.g., give a sum of money for a letter of indulgence, a church-building or similar, regardless of one's character. Without any doubt, this was an erroneous concept. So-called good deeds were not really good deeds. For what derives from a lack of character [Gesinnungslosigkeit] or even an evil character [üble Gesinnung] cannot be called good. Such deeds are customarily called dead deeds. Dead deeds were a sin against the spirit of the Christian religion, as it was especially prevalent in the Middle Ages. An outward church-as-habit [Gewohnheitskirchentum] was the consequence.

Luther and his *Reformation* movement fought against this type of sin. Rightfully he said: action without character [Tun ohne Gesinnung], i.e. deeds without faith, are nothing. Character and faith alone are what counts. Luther in no way wanted to say that the deeds of people do not matter, or that humankind has no ethical duties. It was not necessary to address this, as it is self-evident: Just as genuine character intent, so will faith influence every action. Therefore it is important, that faith is there. This emphasis on faith was very important, as it exposed the wrongs of Middle Age piousness, i.e. dead deeds, and called for their avoidance. Thus, that erroneous course was blocked, indeed.

However, over time another error emerged into the opposite direction. The opinion, that faith has neither influence nor need to influence deeds, became accepted. That proved the most comfortable yet: One need not care about anything, need to feel no restraints in one's actions, and therefore had excuses for others and oneself: "Since deeds do not matter, faith only counts, and that I have". Whoever said this, forgot that such a faith – if he, who pretends this, really should have any – is really not a truly faithful. An intention which will not lead to actions, or at least to an honest try, is not true in itself. Whereas the religious lives of the Middle Ages had dead deeds, the times after Luther suffered from a dead orthodoxy, i.e. a dead orthodox faith attitude [Rechtsgläubigkeit]: "What good is it, though someone say, he has faith, and yet – no works? – Even so faith, if it has no works, is dead, being alone." (James 2:14a, 17). Also here an outward church-as-habit [Gewohnheitskirchentum] followed. It must be emphasized that this erring had nothing to do with Luther's teachings. But it happened and the situation became worse than what had been fought and overcome before. Any action, which lacks character intent, is a doubtful thing. Nevertheless, it is something palpable and may eventually be useful in a practical sense. But a character attitude – or rightly: an imagined character attitude – without actions or at least a willingness to act is empty talk, if not lying, and in any case useless. (A simile: When orders of a state, which do not meet with the approval of its citizens, are followed only because it is required then such an attitude is regrettable, but may be tolerable in extremis. However, it would be most unacceptable, if someone, expressing his free and joyful consent, would not even make an attempt to follow those orders.)

The above described dead faith and pursuant outward church-as-habit caused reactions on many sides in the 18th century – but not a relapse to the old mistake, which Luther had uncovered and fought. The *Pietists* have to be named first. (A.H. Francke and his foundation in Halle, Zinsendorf and the community of the Herrnhut Brethren are also known by non-theologians). *Methodists* appeared in protestant language regions [Sprachregion]. Pietists demanded, instead of a "dead" faith, a "living" faith associated with a pious Christian walk. It was called consecration [Heiligung]. Consecration means in other words, that one believed a real life faith cannot exist without an impact on life-style and actions. The consecration movement lent new life to the Christian walk. At approximately the same time, but from a different mentality the German *Enlightenment* [Aufklärung] followed the same direction. As an example a few lines of Gellert's poem "The active Faith" [Der tätige Glaube]:

"Whoever does not *keep* God's word
and says: I know God! he deceives.

– –

Only then do I please God,
when I practice *obedience*.

– –

A daily active Christianity
is faith's fruit and glory."

This is a reflection of enlightenment in religion, which highly values the practical-ethical side of Christianity, not unlike the sanctification of the Pietist's, demanding "virtue". (Sanctification and virtue are comparable, without being equal: Both stress deeds in contrast to dead faith.)

Also, thoughts and ideas emerged as a reaction to dead faith outside Christian concepts of faith. *Kant* was previously mentioned in the beginning of this article: when he says the will alone is good, it means: all depends on the heart and intent. As intent is characterized by will, action unmistakably is the aim. In the Categorical Imperative Kant admonishes clearly to do good (see above!). Besides, when he discusses the "maxim" of actions, it reveals that, as is necessary, he did not forget the importance of good intent, not repeating the mistakes of the Middle Ages before Luther's time.

Next to Kant and in this context *Goethe* needs mention. At the end of "Faust", part 2 this word is indicative: "Whoever strives and works hard, we can save him." Firstly: The intent [Gesinnung] is what counts. In striving and acting it moves into the realm of the will and clearly aims at deeds. It is interesting to note the similarities of Goethe's words to those of Wesley, the founder of the Methodists, long before: "Do not forget: the reward will be according to your work, not

according to your success." Goethe places decided emphasis on deeds in Faust's great monologue in the 1.part of the tragedy: "In the Beginning was the Deed". These words have remained an uncontested milestone for human conduct, also for the Christian consciousness[1].
Schleiermacher, the most well-known theologian since Luther, validated these insights and discussed the concept of sanctification (proving faith being effective in life) very positively and made it part of his theological teachings[2].

Over time, the situation has changed for the better. As one might say, Catholics do learn from Protestants. However that may be, it appears that some of what the churches were accused of in the Middle Ages has now been remedied, if not removed. Likewise the Protestants have abandoned the erroneous path of dead faith in favor of a living faith. In other words: Man is working in the direction of a Christianity of life and deed. May this way more and more become the only way.

Glauben und Werke in ihrem Gegensatz und in ihrer Vereinigung. *Ethik. Ethik. Sexual- und Gesellschaftsethik. Organ des Ethikbundes,* 1935, 12(6): 260-265

[1] Cf. in this context: Abderhalden in "Ethik" 12(4), p. 151 "If I could as I would like to, then I would underline, what is basic, i.e. the Christianity of Deeds."
[2] Schleiermacher ,"Der Christliche Glaube", paragraph 110-112.

THREE STAGES IN LIFE. 1938

A Contemplation following 2. Corinthians 5:1-10 and the Apostolic Creed

Much in philosophy (Weltanschauung) leads back to the Bible. This fact is quite often forgotten. And so it was with Gustav Theodor *Fechner's* (1801-1887) – scientist and philosopher – little book "Büchlein vom Leben nach dem Tode" [Booklet on Life after Death] (1866). We find exactly the same thoughts in the "Great Didactics" [Grosse Unterrichtslehre] (completed 1657) by Johann Amos *Comenius* (1592-1670), the well known pedagogue and upright Christian and confessor – he was Bishop of the Bohemian Brethren, a branch of the Herrenhuter Brüdergemeinde. Both Fechner and Comenius subdivide human life into three stages. Of special interest is the stage that goes beyond what we know as "this life" to a "life after death", i.e. the stage not only representing the last, but also the commonly acknowledged highest step.

There was one other – long, long before Fechner and Comenius – who perceived the division of human life into three parts, emphasizing the "life after death": it is the apostle *Paul*. It is to Samuel Keller's credit, that he addressed these three stages anew in his book, "Das Los der Toten" [The Lot of the Dead], earlier titled "Auferstehung des Fleisches" [Resurrection of the Body], published after the war of 1914-1918.

Our consideration will focus on the sayings of Paul in 2. Corinthians 5:1-10. These correspond to the three stages of the life of Jesus, as does the Apostles' Creed. These stages are as follows:

First Stage

In the beginning life exists in the "*earthly house*" of the body [*in der Hütte*] (2. Cor. 5:1) (also 2. Peter 1:13, 14) in the terrestrial housing (2. Cor. 5:2) – in the very beginning even in the earthly housing of the mother's body "in flesh" [im Fleische] (Gal 2:20; Phil 1:24; Col 2:1). The first stage in life is a preparation for the second (and lastly also the third). "For we were not placed in this world for nothing, here we must ripen for another" (Matthias Claudius).

Jesus also had to live in an earthly hut and the motherly housing. He took on flesh and blood (John 1:14a) "He was made in the likeness of men: and being found in fashion as a man, he humbled himself" (Phil. 2:7). The Creed speaks of the latter part of his purely human life: ***"Suffered under Pontius Pilate, was crucified, dead and buried"***.

Second Stage

Man is **"*unclothed*"** (2. Cor. 5:4), or he is "absent from the body" (2. Cor. 5:8). It must be noted: To be unclothed does not in all cases mean to be stark naked. To follow the apostle's turn of speech – one can undress short of the undershirt, be in nightclothes and commonly is considered not dressed. Even if completely naked and bare one cannot shed one's skin (also a type of dressing). Upon laying down the mortal form, there may be an "inter-body" [Zwischenleib] or "spirit-body" [Seelenleib], (expressions used by Keller).

With disappearance of earthly clothing, bodily weakness and imperfections disappear as well; Paul considers the release from this body to be liberation. (Romans 7:24)

This state or place of "being unclothed" is the middle stage and may well be called "inter-place" [Zwischenort], "inter-reign" [Zwischenbereich], or "inter-world" [Zwischenwelt]. The New Testament (in the original Greek) calls it "Hades", a word that could also be translated as underworld, world of the dead, world of the departed, shadow-world, soul world or spirit world. The conditions of that in-between world will correspond to how diligently we tried to please God (2. Cor. 5:9), how we lived in this life-body, be it good or evil (2. Cor. 5:10). We might find a state of rest (Rev 14:13), likened to sleep (1. Cor. 11:30, 15:20; 1. Thes. 4:13-15). If this going-to-sleep should signify death, and, if the word death is actually used, then it always refers to a state that shall end in awakening or resurrection. Besides, this condition does not preclude the hearing of Jesus' voice. (Joh. 5:25; 1. Peter 4:6), – Or we find that the spirit-world could become a prison for us (1. Peter 3:19), or a place of torment (Lukas 16:23,24) – named "Tartarus" (2. Peter 2:4 in the original Greek and Latin). Finally a place of blessedness may await us: "Abraham's bosom" (Luke 16:22), a "paradise", an "Elysium", which "no eye has seen, nor ear heard, neither have entered into the heart of man, the things which God has prepared for them that love him" (1. Cor. 2:9), a close communion with Jesus Christ, in contrast to the "Tartarus", mentioned in Peter's 2. Letter. We remember the words of Jesus on the cross. "Verily, I say unto thee, today thou shalt be with me in paradise". (Luke 23:43). The apostle Paul looked forward to that same communion with Jesus: "I desire to depart to be home with the Lord" (2. Cor. 5:8; also Phil 1:23). We share this expectation and ask in song:

"Let go of me, let go of me,
that my Jesus I may see!
My soul is full of longing
to embrace him forever

and to stand before his throne."
(Gustav Friedrich Ludwig Knak).

Johann Hermann's song "Oh God, you faithful God" should also be mentioned here, the 7th verse:
"Take my soul to you
Upward unto your gladness".

How did Jesus fare when he was disrobed of his body? The Creed states: "He ***descended into hell.***"

This is a difficult statement, even for believers: Is not hell the place of eternal damnation and what would Jesus be doing there? Now, Jesus was not really in "'hell'. This word appears only in the German translation of the Creed. In the deciding other-language experience it speaks of under-world, the world of the departed, or shadows, of the souls and spirits, as mentioned above. According to the scriptures and the Creed he was there from Good Friday afternoon to Easter Sunday morning and preached the gospel to the "dead" (1. Peter 4:6), and to "the spirits in prison" (1. Peter 3:19).

Third Stage

Man has been ***"layer-dressed"*** *(überkleidet)* (2 Cor 5:4). The everyday dress is changed into a holiday dress, the hut becomes a palace, the natural body becomes a spiritual and "transfigured" [verklärter] one (Phil 3:21). Whatever is sown in corruption shall rise in incorruption. What is sown in dishonor will rise in glory. What is sown in weakness, will rise in power (1 Cor. 15:42, 43). Looking back we also remember Johann Hermann's song '"O God you holy God", in which the second part of the 7th verse and the 8th contain the prayer:

"In the holy Christian's grave,

do grant the body a place of rest.
On that day, when you will raise the dead,
please extend your hand to my grave
and let your voice be heard,
awaken my body and when resurrected
lead it to the chosen group".

A good summary of the three stages of human life is contained in the liturgy of the Old-Prussian Union [Church] of 1895, and a newer one contains the formulary to be used at funerals: "As it pleased God Almighty to call our brother (sister) from this life (1. Stage), we command his soul to the mercies of God (2. Stage) and lay his (her) body in God's earth – in the hope of a resurrection to eternal life through our Lord Jesus Christ (3. Stage)".

This last mentioned point applies to us all, similar to Jesus, only he already was ***"resurrected on the 3rd day from the dead"***. Eventually the whole world will be transfigured into a new heaven *and a new earth* (2. Peter 3:13; Rev 21:1).

The passage from the first stage to the second is called *"death"*. Naturally this is contrary to the feelings of man. It is tolerated more or less with resignation in silent grief or noisy lament, – just as the baby at birth cries at leaving the mother's protective womb. That is understandable: for leaving your quarters, even if it is only a "hut", is an inconvenience as anyone knows, who has had to move. The laying down of our clothing is also a bit of trouble. Likewise, dying and being born are by nature associated with discomfort, not only the dying itself, but already the thought of it.

Can you not understand the desire to be "layer-dressed" [überkleidet] without removing the other clothes, and "that the perishable could be swallowed up in the new life" without laying down our desires, the hut, the cloth of life? (2. Cor. 5:4; 1. Cor. 15:51-53). According to the Holy Scriptures, Henoch (Gen. 5:24; Heb. 11:5) and Elisha (2. Kings 2:11) were taken up into the kingdom of God without tasting death.

Every Christian hardly dares to share a hope for such special dispensation, but each would like to belong to those who could experience the return of the Lord in this life, they would instantly be "layer-dressed" without being "undressed" before. The apostle Paul anticipated this with great longing (2. Cor. 5:1-4; 1. Cor. 15:51-53). Such longings are in accordance with the Holy Scriptures. "He who testifies to these things says, Surely I come quickly!" (Rev. 22:20) This is answered with the request: "Even so, come, Lord Jesus!" (Rev. 22:20)

But whoever is not called to this immediate passage, will not be far behind those who are. (1. Thes. 4:15) For death, even though appearing to be an end to all life, in reality is only a deliverance from our weakness and imperfection (Rom. 7:24), is the entry-gate to a complete state of being; dying is nothing more than "going home" (2. Cor5:8).

Is not the birth for the child "hard and painful, and death-like for a moment, destroying all previous existence, before the awakening into an outer new being" (Fechner), likewise only a passage into freedom and light?

And what about the kernel of wheat? (cf. 1. Cor. 15:36-38). Does it not appear to be "dead" and get "buried" while being sown? But this dying, being buried and decaying is a mere appearance. In reality the corn swells and sprouts, hidden life-forces stir within it until it rises in a richer form of life than before.

"We mournfully entrust even more precious seed
into the lap of earth,

that from the graves it may bloom
into a happier lot" (Schiller).

From the Christian point of view it is better to use the word 'believe' rather than 'hope': lending it a firm and certain reliance (Heb. 11:1) so that mourning may lose its sharpest thorn.

The two parables of birth and sowing will remind us, that dying always appears like a catastrophic event, – at least for him, who has not yet experienced it before. And this includes all humankind on this earth. But whoever would be able to regard dying in *retrospect*, might perhaps find that it is not such a catastrophe, not nearly as forceful as it *seemed!* In 2. Cor. 5:1 ff., Paul likens dying to a changing of clothes or moving out of a hut, giving a good image: In retrospect, we may find that, when our soul departs our body it may be no more uncomfortable than taking off a coat or clothing, which perhaps were rather uncomfortable and too small and now we feel much better.

It will likely be as if we stepped out of our hut or other building and now stride into a great, free nature. Or as if we exit from a narrow foyer with tarnished windows into a wide and bright hall with unfettered views. And that, in any case, is great improvement.

The passage from the second to the third life-stage is the ***"resurrection"***, "the resurrection of the flesh" (or body) reflected in the third article of the Apostolic Creed. It signifies the redemption of our body (Romans 8:23). To exactly know, how the ascension will occur is not given to us, as we can also not imagine how Jesus arose early on that Easter-morning. But one thing is firm in our faith, that "Christ is risen from the dead, and became the first fruits of them that slept. In him shall all be made alive" (1. Cor. 15:20, 22; 6:14; 2. Cor. 4:14). And "we must all appear before the judgment seat of Christ, so that each one may receive what is due for what he has done in his body, whether it be good or evil." (2. Cor. 5:9, 10). We refer to this in the Creed: Jesus is "*risen to heaven, sitting at the right hand of God, the almighty Father, from whence he will come to judge the quick and the dead*".

Drei Abschnitte des Lebens nach 2. Korinther. *Nach dem Gesetz und Zeugnis. Monatsschrift des Bibelbundes* 1938, 38: 182-188

THE SUNDAY – A SECULAR HOLIDAY. 1947

A Review of Paragraph 10 of the Draft of the Constitution

The work-free Sunday is not at all an achievement of Christian origin. Of course, the Jewish religion had a work-free day. But that was not the Sunday, rather the so-called Shabbat. Christians have observed the Shabbat as long as they lived in Jewish communities. But that was the case only in small Palestine and also for a few decades. Most Christians were Roman citizens and, as such, had no reason to observe a Jewish holiday. And there was no other, no weekly Roman day of rest from work, at least not in the beginnings. That was changed in the year 321 our time: the Sunday was introduced as a work-free day in the Roman Empire. Thus, this day definitely is a governmental, a secular institution.

Secular, therefore, up to today, are the names: Sunday is the day of the sun, – the Romans already named the seven days of the week after the seven planets: Sunday – day of the Sun, Monday – day of the Moon, Tuesday – day of Mars, Wednesday – day of Mercury, Thursday – day of Jupiter, Friday – day of Venus, Saturday – day of Saturn. Since we humans recognize the sun as the largest celestial phenomenon and her eminent importance for all life on earth, it made sense to give the Sunday this very special place among the days of the week.

Something else needs to be considered: Since the sun has been revered in many religions, the Sunday from its beginning had a kind of religious flavor, i.e. a pagan flavor. No wonder: Emperor *Konstantin*, who passed the Sunday law, was a pagan during all his life up to his last hour.

But, of course, the Christians had a great benefit from this day. They could have much more elaborated church services than before. So, for them the Sunday was a real "donatio Constantini", a gift from *Konstantin.*

In summary, the Sunday was an institution of the state regardless of religion and confession. Today it is still the same. See the Constitution of the Weimar Republic, dated August 11, 1919, second part, third section, article 139 "*The Sunday – as a day of rest from labor is protected by law*"". The fact that the day of rest, indeed, was implemented, also is a fruit of the fight of organized labor for their right. Of course, the Sunday was supposed then and also today to be a benefit for Christians. This is indicated by article 139 being a part of the section on religions and churches.

Of actual interest is the 1946 draft of a Constitution for the German Democratic Republic prepared by the Socialist Unity Party of Germany [SED]. In article 16 the Sunday rest is protected by law.[1]

This direction is not so much a response to directions regarding religions and churches, but rather to those protecting the working public. The Sunday is associated with other holidays and with the first of May. In short: It represents itself definitely as a secular holiday, totally consistent with its history.

Thus, the Sunday is not so much a gift from Christianity to the world, rather a gift from the world to all Christians. But the Sunday is not for their exclusive and preferred use, rather for their lawful co-use [Mitbenutzung] (according to arti-

[1] Draft of Constitution, article 16: "The Sunday, other holidays, and May 1 are days of rest and as such are protected by law"

cle 33 of the draft of the Constitution[2]). Everyone without any difference in confession, belief (or unbelief), and weltanschauung may celebrate, whatever one wants to do it: in sport and play, in hiking and walking, in happy companionship, in peace and hobby, in going to church or any other religious activity.

Der Sonntag – ein weltlicher Feiertag. Eine Betrachtung zu Artikel 10 des Verfassungsentwurfs. *Theoretische Zeitschrift des wissenschaftlichen Sozialismus* 1947, 2(6):607-608

[2] Draft of Constitution article 33: "Freedom of belief and conscience and undisturbed practice of religion is protected by the Republic …"

EARLY CHRISTIAN COMMUNIO. 1948

The Communist Manifesto addresses – among other things – an array of socialist systems and experiments, which are based more on literature than reality and are generally of utopian character.

In this regard one may also consider the early Christian Communio, or more precisely: the "Communio Jesu" and its circle of disciples, which today gain a special interest in view of the so-called Christian socialism of today.

One must mention that already more than a hundred years ago *Wilhelm Weitling*, one of the first German socialists, preached about an early Christian communism in his "Gospel of the poor Sinner" [Evangelium des armen Sünders]. Also mentioned should be the writing about Early Christianity [Urchristentum] by *Karl Kautsky*.

To be able to rightly recognize and understand the early Christian Communio, we must occupy ourselves with its founder, with *Jesus* himself. Characteristic for him and his teachings is the section of the Sermon on the Mount, beginning with the sentence: "Lay not up for yourselves treasures upon earth" and ends by saying "Ye cannot serve God and mammon", and much less your possessions, as mammon always and in every case has to be regarded as an unjust mammon.

To the servants of mammon – these are the rich and the proprietors – it is said: "Woe unto the rich, who laugh now, for ye will weep! Woe unto ye, if everyone speaks well of thee!"

These are very radical views and strong expressions, which could be expanded at will. But, how would *Jesus* judge our conditions and practices of business at present: When the profits of an undertaking continually grow, but the worker, necessary to accomplish this gain, receives scanty pay and the buyers of these products must continue to pay exorbitant prices?! When solely for the sake of profit, production is limited, available goods are held back or even destroyed, even though millions of people suffer from great want?! When the blood flows and uncounted people loose life and health, all for the sake of mammon?! And how would the Christian churches of today answer, if in this respect they had kept the spirit of *Jesus*?

Yet what is the reason for *Jesus* position? Why is mammon, wealth, property on the whole, an injustice? We know this from Christ's discussion with the rich man, which we read in the gospels of Matthew, Mark, Luke and in the Evangelium of the Nazaräer. Here he responds to the argument given by the rich man, that he follows God's Laws strictly, with roughly the following: *"How can you assert that? The Law requests: Thou shalt love your neighbor as yourself! But, look now: How many of your folks [Volksgenossen] are dressed in rags, suffer want and are dying from hunger. But your house is full of plenty and nothing ever leaves it!"* – One can see: Jesus was a determined, uncompromising advocate of social justice, of humaneness and compassion, with decidedly religious grounding.

Therefore *Jesus* requested from his followers the renunciation of all private property. He himself acted accordingly: He gave up all personal property. He did not engage in income producing activities and lived from voluntary donations. With his twelve disciples he lived a communal life with truly communal property. After his death they continued their communal life and also accepted many new members into their community. The word community in Greek is „koinonia“, in Latin „communio“. The modern term communism is related to these. Indeed, we may speak about communism among the first Christians.

This Communism is marked by Utopism. The time of *Jesus* and the *Jesus Community* was nowhere near ready for socialist ideas, and even less for their realization. The „Jesus Communio“ was therefore from its beginnings not granted permanence. That it could survive for even some time had religious reasons, in particular the enthusiastic expectation of the imminent return of *Jesus*. Nevertheless, this „Jesus Communio”, the original seed of today’s Christian churches, slowly languished to its end.

Instead, outside of Palestine and in the entire Roman Empire, the Paulinian communities grow, so that *Paulus* became the second, if not the actual, founder of Christianity. Over the centuries these communities grew into the Roman Church, which survived and throve very well even after the collapse of the Roman Empire.

Paulus, who hardly had a relationship with the early Christian [urchristliche] "Jesus Communio" in Jerusalem and no contact whatsoever with the historical *Jesus*, did not seem to have recognized the theory and practice of Communio at all.

Also, one should recognize: Different to *Jesus* and his disciples: *Paulus* was a learned theologian. This is important for the entire following period: The leadership of the church over time came into the hands of theological scholars and clerical officials.

Now, this is the case: Theology and Church are regularly not very open to progress, rather conservative, if not reactionary – specifically in contrast to the laity. i.e. the average people who are not burdened by special interests.

If at all, this is particularly true for the political social sector even more so, because the poor, the very poor, and the average people might not form any longer the basic substance of church membership, but the proprietors, the wealthy, the powerful and their clientele. Of course, the poor were not forgotten. But they became objects of Christian love service, i.e. an organized and private care for the poor, they became recipients of alms [Almosenempfänger].

In the 19th century the time slowly ripened for socialism, and it started not from learned theologians and men of the church rather from the theological laity and people without a church function – just as with Jesus and his community. It did not start from the rich and powerful classes rather it was a movement of the so-called lowest, the working class – as it did before. The founders of modern scientific socialism [wissenschaftlicher Sozialismus] incurred hate and persecution and, if there had been any possibilities, *Marx* and *Engels* might have become liquidated such as *Jesus* at his times.

And the Christian churches today? – Having not delivered what they could or should have, i.e. socialism, they should at least recognize it subsequently. Going with the time, they eventually will. In any case, the appearance of Christian-socialist and religious socialists – and not only recently – may be a symptom for developments into this direction. But, given the hitherto existing traditions, the church will not easily make such a decision.

Pfarrer Fritz Jahr

Urchristliche Communio. *Einheit. Theoretische Zeitschrift des wissenschaftlichen Sozialismus. Herausgegeben vom Parteivorstand der Sozialistischen Einheitspartei Deutschlands*, 1948, 3(3):187-189.

2

Bio-Ethik

Eine Umschau über die ethischen Beziehungen des Menschen zu Tier und Pflanze

Von Fritz Jahr

Die scharfe Scheidung zwischen Tier und Mensch, die seit Beginn unserer europäischen Kultur bis zum Ende des 18. Jahrhunderts herrschend war, kann heute nicht mehr aufrecht erhalten werden. Die Seele des europäischen Menschen rang bis zur französischen Revolution um die Einheit von religiöser, philosophischer und wissenschaftlicher Welterkenntnis, aber diese Einheit haben wir seitdem unter dem Druck der Erkenntnisfülle aufgeben müssen.

Es wird stets das Verdienst der modernen Naturwissenschaft bleiben, daß sie eine vorurteilslose Betrachtung des Weltgeschehens erst möglich gemacht hat. Wir würden uns heute als Wahrheitssucher aufgeben, wenn wir die Erfolge der Tierexperimente, Blutversuche, Serumforschung u. v. a. ablehnen wollten. Andererseits dürfen wir nicht verkennen, daß gerade diese wissenschaftlichen Triumphe des Menschengeistes dem Menschen selbst seine beherrschende Stellung im Weltganzen genommen haben. Die Philosophie, die früher der Naturwissenschaft ihre Leitgedanken vorschrieb, mußte nun selbst ihre Systeme auf naturwissenschaftlichen Einzelerkenntnissen aufbauen, und es war nur eine dichterphilosophische Formulierung der Erkenntnis Darwins, wenn Nietzsche den Menschen als ein recht minderwertiges Übergangsstadium zu einer höheren Entwicklung, als ein „Seil, gespannt zwischen Tier und Übermensch" ansah.

Was folgte aus dieser Umwälzung? Zunächst die grundsätzliche Gleichstellung von Mensch und Tier als Versuchsobjekt der Psychologie. Diese beschränkt sich heute nicht mehr auf den Menschen, sondern arbeitet mit denselben Methoden auch auf dem Gebiet des Tierischen, und wie es eine vergleichende anatomisch-zoologische Forschung gibt, so werden auch höchst lehrreiche Vergleiche zwischen Menschen- und Tierseele angestellt. Ja, sogar die Anfänge einer Pflanzenpsychologie machen sich bemerkbar, — die bekanntesten ihrer Vertreter sind: G. Th. Fechner in der Vergangenheit, R. H. Francé, Ad. Wagner und der Inder Bose in der Gegenwart, sodaß die moderne Psychologie alle Lebewesen in den Bereich ihrer Forschungen zieht. Unter diesen Umständen ist es nur folgerichtig, wenn R. Eisler zusammenfassend von einer *Bio-Psychik* (Seelenkunde alles Lebenden) spricht.

Von der Bio-Psychik ist nur ein Schritt bis zur *Bio-Ethik*, d. h. zur Annahme sittlicher Verpflichtungen nicht nur gegen den Menschen, sondern gegen alle Lebewesen. Sachlich ist die Bio-Ethik durchaus nicht erst eine Entdeckung der Gegenwart. Als ein besonders anziehendes Beispiel aus der Vergangenheit dürfte uns gerade jetzt die Gestalt des hl. Franz von Assisi (1182—1226) mit seiner großen Liebe auch zu den Tieren in der Erinnerung aufsteigen, der in seiner warmen Sympathie für alle Lebewesen der Rousseauschen Schwärmerei für die ganze Natur um Jahrhunderte voraneilte.

Als die Einheit der europäischen Weltanschauung gegen das Ende der Barockzeit zerbrach, war das europäische Geistesleben auch zum erstenmal in der Lage, fremde Gedankenwelten vorurteilslos auf sich wirken zu lassen. Schon Herders umfassender Geist, der für kommende Dinge damals vielleicht die feinste Witterung hatte, erwartete vom Menschen, daß er sich nach dem Vorbild der alles mit ihrem Gefühl durchdringenden Gottheit in jedes Geschöpf versetzen und in dem Maße mit ihm empfinden könne, als das Geschöpf es bedarf. Dieser Gedanke erinnert schon ganz an die indische Geisteswelt, die gerade damals von England aus entdeckt wurde. Aber erst in der Romantik hat Indien das europäische Geistesleben, und seine damals bedeutendste Provinz Deutschland, wirklich befruchtet. Die in Indien ausgebildete Lehre von der Seelenwanderung hat auch das Denken der indischen Philosophenschulen, vor allem der Sankhyaschule beeinflußt. Von dieser Schule trennte sich die Yogalehre ab, die die schärfsten Folgerungen aus diesen Gedankengängen zieht. Der Yogabüßer soll unter keinen Umständen auf Kosten seiner Mitgeschöpfe leben; er soll vor allem keine Tiere töten, aber auch Pflanzenkost nur unter gewissen Voraussetzungen genießen. Er muß ein Tuch vor dem Mund tragen, um beim Einatmen kein noch so kleines Lebewesen zu vernichten; aus demselben Grund muß er das Trinkwasser filtrieren und darf nicht baden. Die Sucht, keinem Lebewesen bei der Selbsterhaltung zu schaden, führt auch noch heute gewisse indische Büßer dazu, sich von Pferdemist zu nähren. Wenn in diesem Zusammenhang natürlich auch Buddha genannt werden muß, so muß doch betont werden, daß gerade von diesem

Religionskünder die fanatischen Selbstschädigungen der Yogaschule abgelehnt wurden. Buddha verbietet den Genuß tierischer Lebensmittel, läßt dagegen Pflanzenkost in weitem Umfang zu. Wie Buddha selbst und seine Lehre vom Glauben der Seelenwanderung durchdrungen war, zeigt für uns Europäer wohl am schönsten die Sammlung der Jatakas, der buddhistischen Märchen, die Buddha in den Mund gelegt werden, und in denen er Geschichten aus seiner früheren Lebenszeit erzählt. Nicht nur als Mensch will er schon gelebt haben, sondern er weiß auch von Daseinsformen zu berichten, in denen er ein Elefant, eine Gazelle, ein Krebs usw. gewesen sein will. Noch schöner als bei Franz von Assisi ist in diesen Geschichten der Gedanke ausgesprochen, daß der Mensch mit allen Geschöpfen wesensverwandt sei.

Diese Gedankenreihen lösten im europäischen Geistesleben seit der Romantik verwandte Gedanken aus, wenn auch natürlich zunächst nicht in dieser schroffen Form. Der Theologe Schleiermacher (1768—1834) erklärte es für unsittlich, daß Leben und Gestaltung, wo sie schon sind, also auch beim Tier und bei der Pflanze, zerstört werden, ohne daß ein vernünftiger Zweck damit verbunden sei. Desgleichen fordert der Philosoph Krause, ein Zeitgenosse Schleiermachers, daß jedes Lebewesen als solches zu achten sei und zwecklos nicht zerstört werden dürfe. Denn sie alle, die Pflanzen und die Tiere, ebenso wie der Mensch, seien gleichberechtigt, allerdings nicht zu gleichem, sondern ein jedes nur zu dem, was ein notwendiges Erfordernis zur Erreichung seiner Bestimmung sei. Offen berief sich auf die indische Gedankenwelt der Philosoph Schopenhauer, der es als einen besonderen Vorzug seiner Ethik ansah, ihre Haupttriebfeder, das Gefühl des Mitleids, auch für das Tier gefordert zu haben. Durch Richard Wagner, der von Schopenhauer stark beeinflußt ist und ein leidenschaftlicher Tier- und Tierschutzfreund war, sind diese Gedanken für breiteste Kreise Allgemeingut geworden.

So ist uns in bezug auf das Tier die sittliche Forderung längst eine Selbstverständlichkeit geworden, wenigstens in der Form, es nicht nutzlos zu quälen. Anders ist es schon mit den Pflanzen. Daß wir auch gegen diese gewisse ethische Pflichten haben, dürfte manchem im ersten Augenblick als widersinnig erscheinen. Aber schon ein Paulus lenkte unser Mitgefühl auch auf Tiere und Pflanzen. Ein Gegenstück dazu sind die verklärt stimmungsvollen Ausführungen im 3. Akt von Richard Wagners Parsifal. In frommer Huld schont der Mensch wenigstens am Karfreitag Halm und Blume auf der Au mit sanftem Schritt, um sie nicht zu verletzen. Aber auch in den pflanzenethischen Überlegungen eines so nüchternen Philosophen, wie es der vor 20 Jahren verstorbene Ed. von Hartmann war, finden wir verwandte Gedanken. In einem Aufsatz über den Blumenluxus schreibt er von einer gepflückten Blüte: „Sie ist ein zum Tode verwundeter Organismus, dessen Farben nur noch nicht beschädigt sind, ein noch lebendes und lächelndes Haupt, das von einem Rumpf getrennt ist. — Wenn ich aber die Rose im Wasserglas oder auf den Draht eines Buketts geflochten sehe, so kann ich mich des widerwärtigen Gedankens nicht erwehren, daß der Mensch ein Blumenleben gemordet hat, damit es im Sterben ein Auge erfreue, das herzlos genug ist, den unnatürlichen Tod unter dem Schein des Lebens nicht herauszufühlen.“

So fein empfindend wie Ed. von Hartmann, ist die große Menge natürlich nicht. Jeder weiß zwar, daß auch die Pflanze ein Lebewesen ist, das durch das Abschneiden der Blumen verletzt wird, aber der Gedanke, daß sie dies auch verspüren könne, liegt uns völlig fern. Soweit ist das Bewußtsein von einer Pflanzenseele noch nicht in uns vorgedrungen. Zudem wissen wir, daß die Blumen auch an der Pflanze selbst verwelken und verdorren, und deshalb findet man an dem Abschneiden von Blumen, namentlich wenn sie zu diesem Zweck herangezogen worden sind, nichts auszusetzen.

Wir gehen dabei von ganz anderen Voraussetzungen aus als die indischen Schwärmer, die überhaupt kein Lebewesen antasten wollen. Auch unsere gesetzlichen oder polizeilichen Bestimmungen über den Schutz einzelner Pflanzen oder Blumen in einer bestimmten Gegend (z. B. der Alpenpflanzen) beruhen auf einer ganz anderen Anschauung: Der Polizeistaat will die betreffenden Pflanzen schützen, damit sie in der Gegend nicht vernichtet werden und später auch noch andere Menschen erfreuen können. Wo eine Pflanze in ausreichender Menge vorhanden ist, denkt der Staat gar nicht daran, sie um ihrer selbst willen zu schützen.

Auch unsere Anschauung vom Tierschutz beruht auf einer wesentlich anderen Grundlage als das Verhalten der Inder. Wenn wir in dem Roman von Richard Voß „Der heilige Haß“ lesen, wie ein Rodyia-Knabe, also ein Angehöriger einer verachteten Kaste, selbst eine giftige Schlange nicht töten will, weil „auch die Schlangen unsere Brüder und Schwestern sind“, so haben wir für dieses Empfinden kein Ver-

4 Fritz Kahn:

ständnis, und wir halten es sogar für unsere Pflicht, schädliche Tiere zu töten, wenn wir können. Wir lassen auch Haustiere vom Schlächter töten oder harmloses Wild vom Jäger erlegen, weil wir Fleisch essen wollen, das manche Leute in unseren Gegenden nicht entbehren zu können glauben, während in tropischen Ländern pflanzliche Nahrungsmittel in überreicher Fülle zur Verfügung stehen. Unser Tierschutz findet also eine Grenze an einem Nützlichkeitsgesichtspunkt, über den sich der Inder kühn hinwegsetzt, und wir begnügen uns damit, wenigstens unnütze Tierquälerei zu vermeiden. Leider reichen noch bei weitem nicht in allen Kulturländern die gesetzlichen Bestimmungen zur Verhütung oder Bestrafung solcher Quälereien aus. Aber wir sind doch auf dem Wege des Fortschritts, und der Tierschutz gewinnt in immer weiteren Kreisen Raum, so wie es ja auch kein anständiger Mensch widerspruchslos ansieht, wenn irgendein Flegel gedankenlos Blumen am Wege mit dem Spazierstock köpft oder wenn Kinder Blumen abreißen, um sie nach wenigen Schritten achtlos wegzuwerfen. Unsere Selbsterziehung hat in dieser Hinsicht schon wesentliche Fortschritte gemacht, aber wir müssen es noch so weit bringen, daß als Richtschnur für unser Handeln die bio-ethische Forderung gilt:

Achte jedes Lebewesen grundsätzlich als einen Selbstzweck, und behandle es nach Möglichkeit als solchen!

Kosmos

Handweiser für Naturfreunde

und Zentralblatt für das naturwissenschaftliche Bildungs- und Sammelwesen

herausgegeben vom

Kosmos, Gesellschaft der Naturfreunde, Stuttgart

24. Jahrgang 1927

POSTSCRIPT

Fritz Jahr (1895-1953) rightly has been called the Father of Bioethics, as we know it. He coined and defined the term Bio-Ethik in 1926 in an article in “Das Mittelschulwesen”, impressed by comparative studies in physiology and psychology in humans, animals and plants by Wilhelm Wundt as well as by philosophical reflections about a potential soul-life of plants by Fr. Th. Fechner and others in the latter part of the 19th century. He transforms and expands Kant’s Catego-rical Imperative into a Bioethical Imperative: “Respect every Living Being on principle as an end in itself and treat it, if possible, as such”. In 1785 Kant only requested respect for “humanity, in your own person as well as in any person, on principle as an end in itself, never only as a means to an end”. “Sanctity of the Moral Law” was the basis for Kant’s Categorical Imperative; for Jahr’s Bioethical Imperative it is “Sanctity of Life”, i.e. compassion with all forms of life and living-together. While Kant’s model was formal and rigorous, Jahr recognizes the interplay between self-care and care for others and replaces the virtue of respect for the law with the virtue of compassion towards all “bios”, i.e. life and all forms of life. Of course, Jahr did not invent the ethics of bios; he refers to European and Asian traditions and gives his 1926 article “The Sciences and the Teaching of Ethics”, describing the function of natural sciences for character formation and the teaching of bioethics, the subtitle “Old Knowledge in New Clothes”.

Jahr’s life was uneventful, marked by poor health and the absence of professional and public recognition during the turbulent times of the Weimar Republic, Fascist Nazi Germany and the Stalinist rule in Eastern Germany. Paul Fritz Max Jahr, child of Gustav Maximilian Jahr, an insurance agent, and his wife Auguste Maria Jahr, nee Langrock, was born January 18, 1895, in Halle (Saale). From 1905 to 1914 he attended the Secondary School of the Franckesche Stiftungen in Halle. In 1913, the Jahr family moved to an apartment in Albert-Schmidt-Str. 8 in Halle, where Fritz would live for the rest of his life. From 1914 to 1921 Jahr studied at the Halle University in Economics, Music, History and Protestant Theology. In November 1920 he passed his teaching exams in Religion and History and in March 1921 he was ordained a Protestant Pastor. He taught at different schools in Halle from 1917 to 1925 and served as Vicar and Assistant Pastor from 1925 to 1932; in 1932 he became Pastor in Kanena near Halle. But already in early 1933 he had to retire due to poor health. The following years, during and after World War II, became quite difficult for him because of poor health and financial constraints. He had married Berta Elise Neuholz in 1932, who died already in 1947 after a long illness wheelchair bound. Fritz Jahr died in October 1, 1953 at the age of 59. In his last years, he resumed private cello lessons to augment his meager pension.

Fritz Jahr did not write voluminous monographs like other original thinkers such as Kant. His publications are short as a good sermon should be, right to the point, ready for practical application and further development by others. Surprising is the breadth and width of his topics ranging from criticism of Esperanto as a formal and static language to that of the hierarchies which he found in churches and elsewhere, from animal ethics and plant ethics to environmental protection and to the recognition that social interactions and communities are not much different from natural biotopes, when individual life depends on give-and-take interaction with others and on good interacting and integrating complexes in struggling for life together. In a translational study to the 5th

Commandment, 1934, he surprises the reader with three steps for the implementation of the 2500 year old rule today: (a) a Golden Rule, (b) good care for one's own health and the health of the family and public health, (c) the Bioethical Imperative. It is not surprising that Pastor Jahr includes in his concept of integrative life also the invisible worlds discussed in religious traditions, – a vision which today can find support in quantum physics and multi-world models.

While Jahr's vision was without any remarkable success in his times, the term Bioethics was re-invented nearly 50 years later by Van Rensselar Potter as the "Science of Survival" (1971). But Jahr had gone further than Potter by including human environments and human bio-topes, such as communities and teams in factories and offices, in his concern for successful and harmonious decision making. There are always informed and educated choices and responsible decisions to be made between self-care and care for others, as he outlines 1929 on the interaction between egoism and altruism.

During the last 40 years the term bioethics unfortunately was quite often used synonymously with the term medical ethics. Most contemporary medical ethics, focusing on respect for patient autonomy and social justice, based on the US Belmont Report (1979) with its emphasis on the three principles of "respect for persons, beneficence, justice", as well as the teachings of the Kennedy Institute of Ethics did not differentiate between "bioethics" and "medical ethics". It was Eve-Marie Engels, who in an article "Bioethik" in Metzler's Lexikon Theologie, 1999, outlined the various branches of bioethics in reference to Fritz Jahr. Hans-Martin Sass published a brochure on "Fritz Jahr's Bioethischer Imperativ" 2007 with the Bochum Zentrum fuer Medizinische Ethik and an article in the "Kennedy Institute of Ethics Journal" 2007, 17: 297-

295. International Conferences in Rijeka (Croatia) 2011 and in Sao Paulo (Brazil) and Halle an der Saale (2012) recently made Jahr's integrative and integrating vision of the "ethics of bios" a prime topic in the development of the foundations of future global bioethics.

This English language edition mirrors the 2nd edition of the Werkausgabe 2013 by Lit Publishers.[1]

I.M.M. H.M.S.

---

[1] Brazilian translations of most of Jahr's publications have been published in "Revista BioEthiKos" 2011, 5(3):242-268; 242-268; Croatian translations by Rinčić, I. and Muzur, A. are in "Fritz Jahr i rađanje europske bioetike" Zagreb: Pergamo 2012. Spanish translations will be published in „Aesthethika" 8(2), 2013; other translations are under way.

INDEX OF NAMES

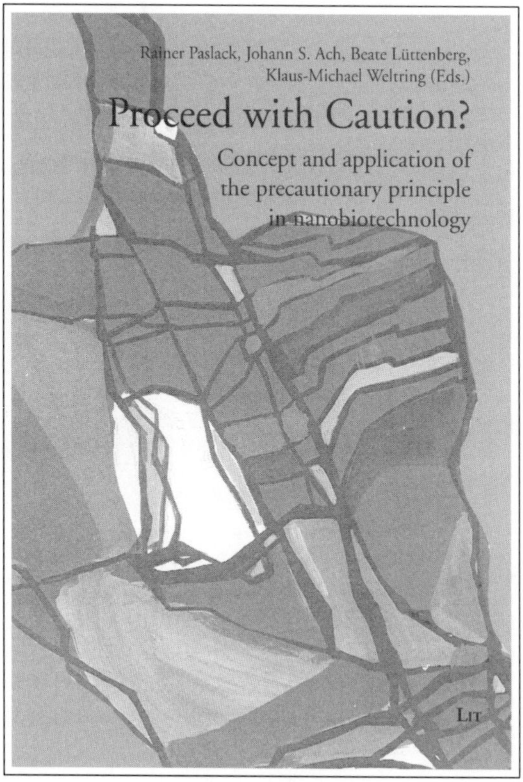

Rainer Paslack; Johann S. Ach; Beate Lüttenberg; Klaus-Michael Weltring (Eds.)
Proceed with Caution?
Concept and application of the precautionary principle in nanobiotechnology
Nanobiotechnology is still a developing field. The results and promises of this technology are not only of scientific and economic importance, they also raise grave ethical, legal and social questions. In this context, especially the so called "Precautionary Principle" or "Vorsorgeprinzip" is of high relevance. What does it mean to "proceed with caution" in the field of nanobiotechnology? How can the principle be applied and specified? Is it a suitable tool for the protection against potentially dangerous effects on the environment and human health? What is the status of the Precautionary Principle in international agreements and national legislation?
Münsteraner Bioethik-Studien, vol. 12, 2012, 248 pp., 29,90 €, br., ISBN-CH 978-3-643-90091-3

LIT Verlag Berlin – Münster – Wien – Zürich – London
Auslieferung Deutschland / Österreich / Schweiz: siehe Impressumsseite